Relationship Counselling with Autistic Neurodiverse Couples

from the same authors

The Autism Couple's Relationship Workbook, Second Edition
Maxine Aston
Foreword by Tony Attwood
ISBN 978 1 78592 891 8
eISBN 978 1 78592 892 5

Neurodiverse Relationships
Autistic and Neurotypical Partners Share Their Experiences
Joanna Pike with Tony Attwood
Foreword by Tony Attwood
ISBN 978 1 78775 028 9
eISBN 978 1 78775 029 6

of related interest

Armchair Conversations on Love and Autism
Secrets of Happy Neurodiverse Couples
Eva A. Mendes
ISBN 978 1 78775 913 8
eISBN 978 1 78775 914 5
audiobook ISBN 978 1 39980 422 6

The Autistic Survival Guide to Therapy
Steph Jones
Forewords by Tony Attwood and Sarah Hendrickx
ISBN 978 1 83997 731 2
eISBN 978 1 83997 730 5
audiobook ISBN 978 1 39981 241 2

Relationship Counselling with Autistic Neurodiverse Couples

A GUIDE FOR PROFESSIONALS

Tony Attwood and Maxine Aston

Foreword by Eva A. Mendes

Jessica Kingsley Publishers
London and Philadelphia

First published in Great Britain in 2025 by Jessica Kingsley Publishers
An imprint of John Murray Press

I

Copyright © Tony Attwood and Maxine Aston 2025

A CIP catalogue record for this title is available from the
British Library and the Library of Congress

ISBN 978 1 80501 302 0
eISBN 978 1 80501 303 7

Printed and bound in Great Britain by TJ Books Limited

Jessica Kingsley Publishers' policy is to use papers that are natural, renewable
and recyclable products and made from wood grown in sustainable
forests. The logging and manufacturing processes are expected to conform
to the environmental regulations of the country of origin.

Jessica Kingsley Publishers
Carmelite House
50 Victoria Embankment
London EC4Y 0DZ

www.jkp.com

John Murray Press
Part of Hodder & Stoughton Ltd
An Hachette Company

The authorised representative in the EEA is Hachette Ireland,
8 Castlecourt Centre, Dublin 15, D15 XTP3, Ireland (email: info@hbgi.ie)

FSC
www.fsc.org

MIX
Paper | Supporting
responsible forestry
FSC® C013056

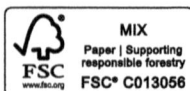

Dedicated to the late Karen Rodman

Contents

Foreword

Navigating the complexities of neurodiverse relationships requires both expertise and empathy. In *Relationship Counselling with Autistic Neurodiverse Couples*, Tony Attwood and Maxine Aston provide one of the most comprehensive resources for understanding and supporting neurodiverse couples in their relational dynamics. As a couple's counsellor with years of experience working with autistic neurodiverse couples from diverse backgrounds, I can confidently say this book reflects the challenges and strengths I see in my own practice.

One of the most common stories I hear from neurodiverse couples is how they've worked with multiple couple's counsellors who either missed the fact that their partner was autistic or failed to understand the unique issues caused by their differing neurologies and provide meaningful guidance to help get their relationship back on track. The lack of autism-informed relationship counselling often leaves couples feeling misunderstood, invalidated and hopeless about improving their connection. Tony and Maxine's work addresses this gap by providing a specialized framework that acknowledges and respects neurodiversity while offering actionable strategies to strengthen relationships.

Drawing on years of research and clinical work, Tony Attwood and Maxine Aston highlight key patterns I've observed in my own practice with autistic neurodiverse couples. While each relationship is unique, common challenges – such as communication barriers, sensory sensitivities, emotional disconnects and societal pressures – often arise. By addressing these core issues in each chapter, Tony and Maxine offer practical counselling strategies, tools and insights on avoiding common pitfalls to help couples strengthen their connections.

Tony and Maxine demonstrate how counsellors can bridge autistic neurodiversity gaps by fostering shared practices that honour both partners' needs. This approach leads to positive counselling outcomes, such as increased understanding, education, improved communication, empowerment and diagnosis – critical to having couples feel that counselling is propelling them in a positive, forward direction. They also thoughtfully address the societal context of neurodiverse relationships, noting how many couples feel pressured to conform to neurotypical relationship norms, often with less-than-ideal outcomes. By promoting a strengths-based approach, Tony and Maxine empower couples to recognize and appreciate the unique contributions each partner brings to the relationship, shifting focus from deficits to strengths.

The book includes research data from neurodiverse couples worldwide, providing a universal context for the strategies presented. This global perspective underscores the effectiveness of the practical recommendations across cultures, making them adaptable and relevant. Tony and Maxine also emphasize the importance of recognizing the individuality of each couple's experience, urging counsellors to adopt a personalized approach that considers neurotype, personality and life experiences. This philosophy aligns with my own practice, where I aim to meet couples where they are and tailor support to their unique needs.

Tony and Maxine recognize the unique challenges counsellors face when working with autistic neurodiverse couples, emphasizing the importance of setting boundaries and practicing self-care. They recommend strategies such as offering extended counselling sessions beyond the standard 50-minute timeslot, having sessions at regular intervals for accountability and assigning concrete homework – approaches I've found essential in my own work. They also provide a checklist for concluding therapy and guiding clients forward.

Blending academic research with clinical practice, *Relationship Counselling with Autistic Neurodiverse Couples* provides a roadmap for counsellors working with these couples. Ultimately, this book calls on couple's counsellors to adopt a beginner's mindset, challenge their notions of neurodiversity and what that can look like in autistic relationships, expand their understanding of autism, take a balanced approach to both the neurotypical and autistic partner's perspectives, and support these couples through empathy and personalized care.

Eva A. Mendes, author of *Armchair Conversations on Love and Autism* and *Marriage and Lasting Relationships with Asperger's Syndrome (Autism Spectrum Disorder)*

Acknowledgements

We would like to thank all the respondents who took the time to reply to our survey and share their experiences of counselling with us. Without your input, this book would not have been possible. This book is written for you and all neurodiverse couples who need support from relationship counselling services.

Maxine would like to offer a special thank you to her daughter Zoe for reading through the chapters and making valuable suggestions based on her own work as a therapist.

Maxine would also like to thank her whole family for their constant support in her writing throughout the past 25 years.

Tony would like to thank his family for their support while writing this book and his colleagues, especially Michelle Garnett, with whom he has developed relationship counselling experience and designed a relationship programme for neurodiverse couples.

Terminology

The terms autistic or non-autistic have been used throughout the book to conform to the present terminology used at the time of publication.

The term autistic includes individuals who have previously had a diagnosis of Asperger's syndrome or 'high functioning autism'.

The statements from the respondents used in this book are all labelled by either AMP or AFP. The former stands for autistic male partner and the latter autistic female partner. The non-autistic respondents are identified by the label NAMP or NAFP which represents non-autistic male partner or non-autistic female partner.

Within the statements quoted from the respondents, references are made to Asperger's, Asperger's syndrome, AS, on the spectrum and ASD. All these would now be referred to as autistic. We have not changed the words and language used by the respondents.

This book is written for all neurodiverse couples regardless of sexuality or gender identification.

Introduction: The Background and Reasons for the Study

When we first discussed the idea for this research in 2014, we had no idea where it would lead, how many responses we would get and what the outcome would be. We were, however, both aware of the large number of negative reports we had received from neurodiverse couples about how let down they felt by the relationship counselling they had received.

These reports regarding their experiences of relationship counselling came from both the autistic partner and the non-autistic partner, some of which were genuinely concerning. For example: one autistic gentleman attended relationship counselling with his non-autistic wife. In the first session the counsellor, who advertised her expertise in working with neurodiverse couples, asked him 'How long have you been affected by this disease?' Following this, the couple walked out of the session, and both were left feeling let down and very disappointed.

Another example was a non-autistic woman being asked by the relationship counsellor why she could not accept that her autistic partner was 'just behaving like a man'. This damming statement, she felt, played a key role in why they gave up as a couple, separated and are now divorced.

These are just two of many examples that we have been privy to, and part of the reason why we decided to discover for ourselves what the experiences of neurodiverse couples who had attended relationship counselling were. We wanted to know first-hand what had worked for couples and what had not worked. We wanted to hear in the couples' own words their experience of relationship counselling and to receive feedback on the all-important question, 'How could current relationship counselling be improved when one of the partners is autistic?'

It is with this in mind that we wrote this book, and it is our hope that both counsellors and counselling organizations will act on the information and advice that it contains. This book is to give voice to all the couples that have been let down by the counselling support they received and as a consequence have had their relationship damaged by the outcome. The evidence from our survey indicated very strongly that relationship counselling failed because the counsellor did not recognize that the couple were neurodiverse or because they had not received adequate training to understand and work in this area.

We both hope that this book will play a part in changing this shortfall in relationship counselling and neurodiverse couples will be offered the understanding and support they so greatly require.

SECTION ONE

The Research Survey

The authors would like to note that the results from this survey do not represent all neurodiverse couples; they represent couples who have required the support and services of a relationship counsellor and should not be generalized to all neurodiverse couples.

CHAPTER 1

The Respondents to the Survey

To validate the research, we asked for two prerequisites to be fulfilled for the individual's response to be included in the research/survey. These were:

1. The respondent must have attended relationship counselling with their partner.

2. The respondent must either be autistic or they must be the partner of an autistic individual.

We posted the link and information regarding the research on our websites, taking time to explain exactly what the purpose of the research was. (See Appendix 1 for the complete questionnaire.)

Responses to our research began to come in, and we kept the research live until 2021, when we both considered that we had accumulated enough data for analysis. The total number of completed questionnaires we received was 225. This number consisted of 184 questionnaires from non-autistic individuals whose partner had received a diagnosis of autism, and a further 41 questionnaires from individuals who identified as autistic. For full details of respondents' ages, nationalities and occupations see Appendixes 2 and 3.

Some interesting patterns emerged from the respondents' occupations. Teaching and counselling ranked highest for the non-autistic partner, whereas engineering and IT ranked highest for the autistic partner.

It is not unusual for autistic individuals to find employment that involves their special interests. Tony discussed this in his book *The Complete Guide to Asperger Syndrome* first published in 2006. Tony describes how autistic individuals are able to become experts and excel in their particular field of interest and will be able to talk and discuss with confidence the interests they hold.

Of the 40 non-autistic women, 23% worked in the caring profession, working as either counsellors, therapists, nurses or carers, and a further 19 respondents described themselves as homemakers or mothers. The teaching profession (23) accounted for 13% of the respondents. These results strongly back our speculation regarding the often sociable, caring and empathetic nature of many of the non-autistic women who find themselves in a relationship with an autistic man.

Only four non-autistic men responded to our survey; two did not supply any information regarding their career choice. The two that did were working in IT and education. Therefore, it is not possible to say whether the non-autistic male partners would be more likely to be working in the caring and teaching professions.

Another difference found between the couples was that in 31 of the relationships, the partners came from different countries of origin. It was noted, in addition, that for 14 of these couples, their countries of origin had a different national language. This could in some cases suggest that the couple did not share the same first language, which may have disguised communication difficulties caused by a neurological difference.

One explanation for the diverse mixture of cultures could be that many of the relationships were the outcome of online dating. Meeting a partner over the internet can offer a safe haven for an autistic adult and provide a less stressful and more hopeful setting than face-to-face dating (Roth & Gillis, 2015). Online dating eases many of the social demands involved in trying to build a rapport with another individual. It also offers far more choice and variety of possible romantic connections, as these are not limited by location. Dating this way offers autistic adults better control and more processing time to consider their responses and greatly reduces the constant need to interpret non-verbal cues (Roth & Gillis, 2015). Roth and Gillis in 2015 found that 53% of autistic adults used online dating compared to 15% in the general population (Smith, 2016).

We did not enquire in our research as to how couples initially met, and there is little or no research that has studied whether either compatibility is increased or communication is easier when culture and language are different in neurodiverse relationships. It is certainly very possible that, due to the increased use of online dating, the chances of the autistic individual meeting someone from a different country are higher.

The questionnaire asked what were the positives and negatives that respondents believed they derived from attending couple counselling. In the next chapter, we will start by exploring the feedback provided by the autistic respondents. We will look at the positives, followed by the negatives. In the following chapters, we will continue by exploring the positives and negatives provided by the non-autistic sample.

REFERENCES

Attwood, T. (2006). *The complete guide to Asperger's syndrome*. Jessica Kingsley Publishers.

Roth, M. E., & Gillis, J. M. (2015). 'Convenience with the click of a mouse': A survey of adults with autism spectrum disorder on online dating. *Sexuality and Disability, 33*, 133–150. https://doi.org/10.1007/s11195-014-9392-2

Smith, A. (2016). *15% of American adults have used online dating apps or mobile phone dating apps*. Pew Research Center. www.pewresearch.org/wp-content/uploads/sites/9/2016/02/PI_2016.02.11_Online-Dating_FINAL.pdf

CHAPTER 2

The Autistic Partner's Perspective on the Positives of Couple Counselling

The group of autistic partners consisted of 25 men and 16 women who had either been formally diagnosed or self-diagnosed, as in the case of three men and two women.

Three women and one man identified their partner as also being on the spectrum, and one man identified as being in a homosexual relationship with a non-autistic man.

In the questionnaire, Question 8 asked 'What was the most useful aspect of the counselling?'

Question 10 asked 'Do you believe the counselling had a positive effect on the relationship?' If the answer was yes then Questions 11 and 12 asked 'If yes, what were the positive effects on yourself?' and then 'your partner?'

A total of 41 individuals identified as autistic responded to the survey. As some of the respondents had attended couple counselling on more than one occasion, this resulted in 57 couple counselling cases.

Reading through the responses to the questions above, only 15 out of a possible 57 cases were reported as leading to an overall positive outcome for the couple. Importantly in almost all the positive outcomes the counsellors were aware that the couple were neurodiverse and had received some form of training on autism.

The positives that respondents felt they had received from the counselling fit into five groups:

- Increased understanding

- Education

- Improved communication

- Empowerment/validation

- Diagnosis.

All these groups are strongly related and interwoven. In many cases, one group leads to another and is clearly correlated. For the sake of clarification in this chapter, we will explore each group of positive outcomes individually, starting with understanding.

INCREASED UNDERSTANDING

An increased understanding of their self, partner and relationship was expressed as a key benefit from the couple counselling attended by the autistic participants in the survey. One autistic man stated, 'I understood myself better', whilst an autistic woman stated 'It [couple counselling] was very helpful to give us both a lot more understanding'.

The fact that couple counselling had helped both the autistic respondents and their partners to understand each other better was given as a positive in the survey. In romantic relationships, feeling understood by one's partner is crucial in forming and maintaining an intimate relationship. Feeling understood builds trust in one's partner and allows for closeness and connectedness, giving a sense of belonging in a relationship. Feeling understood has also been found to correlate with feeling healthy and happy (Lun et al., 2008).

One of the roles of a couple counsellor is to build a relationship with their clients that is honest and empathetic; for empathy to be sincere, the counsellor must have a genuine understanding of their client and their client's internal frame of reference, regardless of what form that takes.

The couple counsellor having an understanding of the effects of autism in a relationship can, at this vulnerable and fragile stage in their clients' relationship, make the difference between a couple staying together or not.

In the group with positive outcomes, 12 of the 15 couple counsellors involved were aware of the presence of autism, and 10 of these 12 had received some training in the effects of autism and were able to offer understanding for both the autistic client and the non-autistic client. The feeling of being understood by the therapist is evident in the statements that respondents used to describe their counselling experience. For example:

> (AMP) 'My partner felt like someone else was on our side and understood her, which reduced the pressure on her, and the counsellor helped her to understand me'.

> (AMP) 'Feeling understood by the therapist'.

Feeling understood by a professional will help reduce the fear and uncertainty of the couple. For the autistic client, hearing a third party that they trust describe in a way that is logical and unbiased the reasons for the difficulties being faced in the relationship can come as a revelation. Hearing from a third party is far more likely to be accepted and understood by the autistic client than being told by their non-autistic partner, as the third party will, hopefully, be perceived as unbiased. Being understood by another can restore confidence and trust and build self-esteem. This will provide a way forward for a couple to make progress, as was expressed by one woman who stated:

> (AFP) 'I understood more what was happening and what I could do to improve the relationship'.

Being given a better broad understanding of autism can be helpful, if not essential, to both partners. Based on this, it is not surprising that being offered accurate and useful information and education from the couple's counsellor ranked second in the positives that the autistic partner felt they received from the counselling.

EDUCATION

Once a clear understanding that one (or both) of the clients are autistic is established between the counsellor and the couple, the next important step is for the counsellor to be able to educate both partners on what this actually means for them and their relationship.

The counsellor must have a thorough understanding of autism and especially what, in the relationship, is due to misunderstanding autism and what is due to personality differences. The counsellor will be educating the non-autistic partner on the effects of being autistic.

The counsellor should be able to offer suggestions and ideas that could improve communication and work towards developing a more neuroaffirming, intimate and realistic relationship.

As with the non-autistic partner, the counsellor will also be educating the autistic partner on what it means to be non-autistic and why things such as emotional reciprocity, intimate conversations and sharing quality time together may be important to the non-autistic partner.

The counsellor's role as an educator is enormous and must fulfil very large criteria as there will be so many areas in the relationship to cover. This will start with the development of a basic understanding of what autism is. The learning process may take time and practice. The counselling will be seeking to help the couple change and improve the underlying structure and foundations of the couple's relationship. The development of couple and family harmony, replacing unrealistic expectations with achievable ones, is paramount to the success of the therapy. If children are involved, the changes must also include and benefit them.

Respondents highlighted many areas in which they believed their relationships had benefited from the knowledge of the couple counsellor. Here are some examples:

(AMP) 'She [my partner] learned why I do what I do'.

The above example shows how simply understanding autistic traits and the autistic experience within a neurotypical world can be felt as a benefit to a relationship. For many couples, by the time they attend counselling together, years of misunderstandings may have accumulated, years of making assumptions with no knowledge of how to respond or make workable improvements to the relationship. Without understanding and education, it is almost impossible for a neurodiverse couple to go forward, and this is strongly highlighted in the comment below:

(AMP) 'I learned many behaviours I need to improve'.

Respondents learnt what they could do to make improvements to benefit the relationship. This knowledge could, for some, increase the feelings of being in control and empowered. This is very important for both mental health and self-esteem. Equally, the respondents commented on how the learning had benefited their non-autistic partners:

(AFP) 'Husband learned that my behaviour was not always about him, [it is] the environment causing me to feel overwhelmed'.

Sensory sensitivity affects many (but not all) autistic individuals and this is an area that the counsellor will need to explore with the couple. If an autistic individual does have some areas in which they are sensitive this can, without awareness or understanding, prove quite confusing for the non-autistic partner, especially when it has a negative effect on intimacy and physical closeness.

For the non-autistic partner, it might be learning that their autistic partner is not being rude or detached if they, for example, refuse to share their mealtime with the family. The reason could be due to finding specific noises, such as the sound of chewing, very distressing. On a more intimate level, the benefit for both might be learning that touching the areas of the body that would be assumed to be pleasurable by the non-autistic partner can be painful to some autistic individuals. This could again be due to hypersensitivity, and counselling should explore, with the couple, any difficulties or concerns in the area of the sexual side of the relationship. Helping the couple to understand that both over- and under-sensitivity are traits of autism and what this means for them and their relationship can be of huge benefit, helping to create understanding and restoring the self-esteem of both. It is all about learning, which without the awareness and understanding of the counsellor is unachievable. Every autistic individual's sensory experience will be different, and various factors, especially stress and anxiety, will contribute to their experience, which can change from day to day.

The respondents in this group of positive outcomes also reported how they had been able to learn strategies and coping skills for both them and their partners from attending couple counselling, as described in the comments below:

(AMP) 'She [counsellor] helped us with exercises, such as thinking about how to trust different people and what to do in certain situations, such as when I was feeling panicked'.

(AFP) 'Strategies to prevent my outbursts/meltdowns or know when or why they would most likely occur'.

When counselling couples where one or both are autistic, the counsellor needs to be trained in the appropriateness and effectiveness of the strategies and skills taught to the couple. Recommending the wrong tools or exercises can result in failure and have a devastating effect on the relationship, as well as the client's self-esteem. These negative effects are discussed more in Chapter 3. As seen, though, from the examples above, the right strategies can make highly beneficial improvements to the smooth running of the relationship and the harmony between the couple.

In the same way that understanding requires learning, understanding and learning also lead to improved communication, which bring us on to our next positive outcome.

IMPROVED COMMUNICATION

Without an understanding of the double empathy problem and acceptance of each other in a relationship, it is almost certain that misunderstandings in communication will follow. Both partners will be working on the misguided assumptions that they have formed over time regarding their partner's personality and behaviour. Lack of knowledge and understanding will have clouded the perceptions of each about the other; this will cause actions and communications to be misinterpreted as criticism, which will trigger a defensive reaction in the other.

One of the primary reasons for the breakdown of communication in an autistic neurodiverse relationship is due to the consequences of the double empathy problem. Misunderstandings in communication have, in the past, been presumed to be due to the autistic partner's lack of empathy and the difficulties they experienced in reading the thoughts, feelings and intentions of others. However, this assumption has now been challenged: research is finding that autistic individuals do in fact feel empathy, but since it is equally difficult for non-autistic people to read the thoughts, feeling and intentions of autistic people, this is frequently misinterpreted. The double empathy problem is the term used to describe this situation (Milton, 2012).

One of the key roles of the couple counsellor is as a translator between the couple, interpreting the true meanings behind the communication shared. The counsellor will teach, by way of example, how to talk in each other's language and to be aware that both partners may be struggling to read each other accurately. This is shown in the quote below:

(AMP) 'She [counsellor] helped us communicate and better understand each other'.

One of the primary reasons that couples seek out the services of couple counselling is because all communication has broken down between them. At its worst, attempts to communicate may have ceased altogether as it may feel that even taking breath can result in the other partner becoming defensive. Trying to communicate has totally failed and one or both partners will have completely withdrawn and will not communicate about anything unless it is totally necessary to keep the household/family running. Absolute stalemate. We have encountered this so often in the counselling room; it is a sensitive situation that can only be changed through understanding and education. Reforming communication can produce outstanding benefits and improvements in how the relationship is managed and how both partners feel about themselves and each other.

This is shown in the quote below:

(AMP) 'The fact that she [counsellor] got us to talk together without arguing'.

Working with a counsellor who has a genuine understanding of how the double empathy problem will affect the couple's ability to read each other accurately is imperative and would undoubtedly be very beneficial to the relationship. For some this understanding was empowering and helped greatly to increase self-awareness and self-esteem.

Other respondents felt that the benefit of the communication in counselling was more personal to them as individuals than the relationship. Some respondents expressed the beneficial effect of simply being listened to by the counsellor or having someone to talk to and feel understood.

EMPOWERMENT/VALIDATION
One of the most basic roles of good counselling is for a counsellor to be able to offer their client complete and genuine unconditional positive self-regard and a safe place for the client to be able to express themselves freely without fear of judgement. This affirming experience will make it possible for the client to feel validated, reassured and will aid in the restoration of the client's self-esteem and self-worth.

Unconditional positive regard, empathy and congruence are believed by Carl Rogers (1957) to be the three core conditions in the therapeutic process needed for change to be achieved.

From the statements about the 15 counselling cases that were reported as being positive, the following two show how receiving these three core conditions in counselling were of benefit:

(AMP) 'She [counsellor] helped me deal with issues...and to feel marginally less of a failure than I ordinarily feel'.

(AFP) 'Validation of what I have achieved, but also what I have sacrificed, through my commitment to our relationship'.

Autism does not compromise intellect. However, autistic individuals can have difficulty 'reading' other people – recognizing others' feelings and intentions – and expressing their own emotions. This can cause confusion and can leave the autistic individual feeling acutely aware that, within the relationship, there is something they are not getting right. Most autistic partners are aware that there is a fundamental emotional need their partner has that, no matter how hard they try, they keep failing to meet. This can leave the autistic partner feeling frustrated that their partner misinterprets their intentions or does not recognize that they are trying very hard to get it right for them. Consequently both partners will be confused, both will feel frustrated and both will be struggling to figure out what they can do to achieve harmony in the relationship and end the feelings of blame and guilt.

Without a counsellor who can offer the three core conditions of unconditional positive regard, empathy and congruence to the couple, neither will feel validated, accepted or understood.

Respondents stated how they felt the counselling offered them confirmation, validation and was affirming. The benefits of this were experienced as greater self-awareness, feeling supported to deal with unresolved issues and being able to reform boundaries within the relationship.

Many of the autistic clients we have worked with have initially come to the couple counselling sessions saying very little, often allowing their partner to talk for them. This is a pattern that can easily evolve in a neurodiverse relationship if there is a history of the autistic partner 'getting it wrong'. The consequence can be total withdrawal and a lack of communicative interaction between the couple.

A counsellor who is able to offer unconditional positive regard to the autistic partner will allow them to feel heard, valued and safe. As a female respondent stated, the counselling 'gave her a voice'.

DIAGNOSIS

We have also included diagnosis as an important benefit that was gained by some respondents from counselling. Unfortunately, there were only four respondents who, as a consequence of couple counselling, discovered that they were autistic. Having a formal diagnosis for some couples is the only way forward, whereas for others, just being self-diagnosed or knowing is enough.

The consequences of a diagnosis can be negative or positive, and this will depend entirely on the nature of both partners in the relationship and most importantly the stage and state of the relationship when autism is discovered.

Being offered awareness and understanding of autism and what it means for both the individual and the couple can be a key factor in a couple's decision to stay together and work to bridge their differences. The role of the counsellor at this sensitive and vulnerable stage for a couple is crucial. If the counsellor is unaccepting of autism and has no training or knowledge in this area it can result in the breakdown of the therapeutic relationship. Research has found the strength of the therapeutic relationship is a factor in successful therapy outcomes, independent of therapeutic approach (Bergin & Lambert, 1978; Martin et al., 2000).

REFERENCES

Bergin, A. E., & Lambert, M. J. (1978). The evaluation of therapeutic outcomes. In S. L. Garfield & A. E. Bergin (Eds.), *Handbook of psychotherapy and behaviour change* (2nd ed.). Wiley.

Lun, J., Kesebir, S., & Oishi, S. (2008). On feeling understood and feeling well: The role of interdependence. *Journal of Research in Personality, 42*(6), 1623–1628.

Martin, D. J., Garske, J. P., & Davis, M. K. (2000). Relation of the therapeutic alliance with outcome and other variables: A meta-analytic review. *Journal of Consulting and Clinical Psychology, 68*, 438–450.

Milton, D. E. M. (2012). On the ontological status of autism: The 'double empathy problem'. *Disability & Society, 27*(6), 883–887. https://doi.org/10.1080/09687599.2012.710008

Rogers, C. R. (1957). The necessary and sufficient conditions of therapeutic personality change. *Journal of Consulting Psychology, 21*, 95–103.

CHAPTER 3

The Autistic Partner's Perspective on the Negatives of Couple Counselling

Question 9 asked, 'What was the least useful aspect of the counselling?'

Question 13 asked, 'Do you believe the counselling had a negative effect on the relationship? If the answer was yes, then Questions 14 and 15 asked, 'If yes, what were the negative effects on yourself?' and then 'your partner?'

Reading through the responses to the questions above, nearly half of the reported 57 cases confirmed an overall negative outcome for the couple. Only one of the counsellors in this group had received any training in autism and this was in working with autistic children, not adults. Although three counsellors in this group claimed to have some knowledge of autism this was disputed by the respondents.

During the counselling sessions, many of the counsellors were informed by the respondents or their partners that it was suspected that one of them was autistic; in one case however this was dismissed by a counsellor.

Respondents who did not report a positive or negative outcome stated that the counselling had no effect or failed to produce any change in the relationship. A small number felt the counselling resulted in a mixture of positives and negatives. Almost all the counsellors involved had not received any training in working with neurodiverse couples.

The negatives that respondents felt they had experienced from the counselling fit into four themes:

- Lack of understanding

- Disempowerment

- Negative effect on emotional well-being

- Relationship deteriorated due to the counselling.

All these negative outcomes are strongly related and interwoven. In many cases, one theme leads to another and is clearly correlated. We will, though, for the sake of clarification in this chapter, explore each theme individually, starting with the lack of understanding that was experienced by the autistic partner in the couple counselling.

LACK OF UNDERSTANDING

Not feeling understood by the therapist was given as a frequent downfall in the counselling experience, as seen in the examples below:

> (AMP) 'Therapist did not understand AS [autism] which made things worse'.

> (AMP) 'The advice she [counsellor] did give showed a lack of understanding of AS'.

Autism is a different way of perceiving, thinking, learning and socially relating to others. Many autistic respondents reported how they had felt that the therapist did not understand them, their partners or, importantly, autism. Autistic clients we have seen have frequently expressed a history of feeling not understood by others. Research is finding that autistic individuals, compared to non-autistic individuals, are often seen in a less favourable light by the non-autistic population (Sasson et al., 2017). Many autistic adults may have grown up with little or no awareness that they were autistic, yet they were acutely aware of feeling different, not fitting in and often, sadly, being excluded by their peers without any knowledge of why. This feeling of being excluded and not being understood by their peers and professionals can lead to low self-esteem and the risk of mental health issues, especially depression (Cassidy & Rodgers, 2017).

It is vital for a counsellor to be able to relate to and empathize with their client's internal frame of reference if the counselling is going to create a relationship based on understanding and trust. However, it was shown that in many of the couple counselling attendances described by the respondents this was not the case. A lack of skills and training to understand the autistic client or their partner may result in a counsellor assuming the couple is non-autistic and thus responding to them from an uninformed perspective.

In a counselling context, counsellors must relate to their client's frame of reference. According to Tudor and Merry (2006, p. 58), an individual's frame of reference is the 'subjective and unique way' in which they understand 'others and the world'. This unique understanding will be based on their perceptions and life experiences. In a therapeutic relationship it is crucial that a counsellor can empathetically understand and respond to their client's frame of reference (internal) and not their own frame of reference (external) (Nelson-Jones, 2009, p. 55).

If this is not achieved and a genuine and empathetic understanding is not offered by the counsellor, then both the clients and the therapeutic relationship will be harmed and will suffer (Brodley, 1999).

In order to fit in with the social expectations of a predominantly neurotypical world, many autistic individuals will have learnt from an early age to camouflage and hide any autistic traits. Learning to mask behaviours, for many autistic individuals, would have been a way of surviving in a world that offered little understanding of what it meant to be autistic. Masking behaviours require a huge amount of mental energy (Hull et al., 2017; Tierney et al., 2016) and can leave autistic individuals feeling drained and vulnerable to depression and anxiety (Gillott & Standen, 2007). Autistic women are particularly at risk in this area as some areas of research have found that autistic women are more likely to take on masking behaviour than autistic men (Lai et al., 2017).

Masking behaviour is most likely to be dominant at the beginning of a relationship when the autistic individual is focused on their chosen partner and has the strong desire to fit in with their needs and form a relationship. Unfortunately, due to the massive amount of mental energy and effort it takes, masking is impossible to maintain long term; trying to do so would have a very negative effect on the autistic individual. Although being able to unmask is essential and healthy, it can involve the autistic individual needing to have their own space and time to pursue their own interests. This, sometimes sudden change in behaviour can appear as withdrawing and becoming detached, and can leave the non-autistic partner confused and unable to understand why their partner is suddenly behaving in such an unfamiliar and seemingly uncaring way.

Equally, the autistic partner may also be struggling to understand why their partner is no longer happy in the relationship and why they now find it so difficult, or even impossible, to make them happy. In a study by Strunz et al. (2017), it was found that 65% of autistic individuals reported feeling fearful that they would not be able to meet or fulfil their partner's expectations. Autistic individuals will be very aware of their partners frequently pointing out to them what it is they are not getting right, or how their words and behaviour, or lack of words and behaviour, are responsible for the upset their non-autistic partner is experiencing. However, without having all the information, this can easily be interpreted by the autistic adult as 'criticism without cause'. This perceived criticism could trigger a defensive reaction in the autistic partner, as they will rarely be aware of what it is they have done to cause upset. Hence, the distance will grow between the couple as they will not be able to resolve the issues and miscommunications that frequently occur between them.

Without any positive intervention, the couple will soon find themselves in a place of no understanding, self-doubt, blaming, guilt and low self-esteem.

This is often the point at which the decision is made to seek the help and guidance of couple counselling, and for some, it is, after many years of misunderstandings and assumptions, the last chance for the relationship to mend and work out.

We have found that it is more likely to be the non-autistic partner who takes the initiative to arrange couple counselling, and it might have been raised many times before the autistic partner agrees to go. In many cases, it is only when the non-autistic partner threatens to leave or end the relationship that an agreement to go to counselling together is finally achieved. We have both observed that some autistic individuals may feel the need to revert to masking behaviour in the counselling room, trying their best to appear calm, pleasant and polite, and often having a desire for the counsellor to like them. Obviously, this will potentially cause frustration and annoyance for the non-autistic partner, who will feel that a true picture of the relationship is not being portrayed in the counselling room.

Unless the counsellor is aware of the presence of masking and autism and has both knowledge and training in the dynamics this can cause in an intimate relationship, they will be totally misguided and misled. They will only be guided by the communication and actions of their client in the room, missing the internal, underlying reasons for the behaviour presented. This would result in the counsellor responding in a way not beneficial to the couple, which could create feelings of mistrust and doubt.

The autistic respondents frequently felt that the counselling was biased against them, favouring the non-autistic partner; however, this was not always the case. One autistic female pointed out how she felt the counsellor focused more on her rather than her non-autistic partner. This in turn negatively impacted her and the relationship, as this was not what she wanted.

> (AFP) 'He [partner] felt helpless without anyone understanding and supporting him... It led to a lot of conflict and misunderstandings with the therapist favouring the ASD partner and not taking care of the non-autistic'.

In couple counselling, the counsellor must offer a balance in the session, not showing a bias towards either partner. There is little research into whether, in couple therapy, a counsellor is likely to be biased towards one particular partner. However, as noted previously, there are many studies emerging that show that autistic individuals tend to be seen in a less favourable light compared to non-autistic individuals by the non-autistic population. This is more likely when the non-autistic individual is not aware that the person in question is autistic, as DeBrabander et al. (2019) found in their study on first impressions. For many of the respondents, neither they nor the counsellor were aware that autism was present. This resulted in a lack of understanding from the counsellor and led to the counselling being ineffective.

If the counsellor does not understand autism and the challenges faced by the autistic partner in the relationship, then the result is that the advice and support being offered will not be effective. Additionally, if this lack of understanding leads to the counsellor giving unachievable and unsuitable exercises and strategies for a neurodiverse couple to practice, then the result is likely to be feelings of disappointment for the non-autistic partner and, as described by one autistic client, couple counselling being a 'A demoralizing experience'.

DISEMPOWERMENT

We have found in our work that for many of the autistic clients we have seen, their main reason for coming to counselling is that they want their partner to be happy, as they are aware that for some reason this is not the case.

It is rarely the intention of the autistic partner to cause upset or unhappiness for their spouse. Their hope in couple counselling is often that a professional will be able to explain this to their partners and help their partners understand them. Their hope is often that the counsellor will be able to give them a voice and put into words what they would like to say. They are often looking for the counsellor to supply the emotional support that their partner states they are lacking.

Feelings of failure in the relationship have often been described by the autistic clients we have worked with, particularly among the male clients. The majority of the autistic clients that attend couple counselling do so because they desperately want to make the relationship work, often with the hope that the counsellor will be able to tell them what it is they are supposed to do and how to do it. Half of autistic adults reported that they did not know how romantic couple relationships worked or how to maintain them (Strunz et al., 2017). If the counsellor does not have a good understanding of what it means to be autistic, it is likely that unrealistic expectations will be put on the autistic partner to be able to complete tasks and exercises designed for a non-autistic relationship.

An exercise frequently used in non-autistic couple counselling is to spend maybe two minutes each evening taking turns talking, uninterrupted, about innermost emotions. For autistic people, and especially for those who also experience alexithymia, which is difficulty expressing thoughts and feelings in words, this exercise and others could prove very stressful and virtually impossible to complete.

(AMP) 'Exercises for me (I had difficulty completing them)'.

(AFP) 'It [counselling] expected of me things I just cannot do'.

Being given unachievable exercises can be very damaging and undermining for the autistic partner and can lead to feelings of disempowerment and low self-esteem. Feelings of disempowerment in the autistic partner will often be exacerbated by the disappointment expressed by the non-autistic partner. By being prescribed these exercises by a professional, the non-autistic partner is likely to have presumed that they were realistic and could wrongly interpret their partner's avoidance or lack of willingness to try as 'not caring enough'. The non-autistic partner's disappointment will increase the autistic partner's feelings of failure.

Due to the invisibility of being autistic in some individuals, coupled with the ability to mask, if the counsellor has not been trained in this area, misjudgements will be made. Without any knowledge that the couple are neurodiverse, the counsellor will not be aware that tasks that include spontaneous emotional communication and expression have the potential to cause significant damage to both partners. The consequences could include increased stress and anxiety in the autistic partner, who may already regard themselves as failing to meet the expectations of both their partner and their counsellor; and the non-autistic client could be left feeling their partner is being uncooperative and not trying to make the relationship work. The counselling will have failed before it even really began, as trust will have been thoroughly broken.

This is clearly expressed in the examples below:

(AMP) 'We never got to the bottom of the issues which I guess were all about Asperger's, this means, for me, that I was kind of forced into a straightjacket to behave in a way I could not. I always felt I was "the bad guy" in these sessions'.

Feelings of being pressured and forced to act, communicate or behave in a certain way were frequently described. For some, the tasks given did not consider sensory issues, which are likely to be experienced by the autistic partner, especially in the physical and sexual side of the relationship, as described by one autistic female respondent below:

(AFP) 'Feeling pressured to engage more physically with my partner'.

Counselling should not at any point leave a client feeling pressured into behaving physically, sexually or mentally in any way that is not agreed to or takes into account what is best for and beneficial to the client. Working with neurodiverse couples requires a thorough understanding of both partners equally. If the counselling is biased towards one partner, it will be detrimental to the couple's relationship. The counsellor is often viewed as the professional, the one who should be guiding the situation, the one who should carry the interests of both partners in perfect balance, without tasks or communication favouring either. It is the counsellor's responsibility to monitor the words they use and how they communicate with their clients so that they do not disadvantage either of them.

Reports from respondents below showed that often, this was not the case:

(AFP) 'Small talk at least 50% of the session'.

(AMP) 'Being expected to be able to participate in a three-way conversation and not being able to express myself well verbally'.

Difficulties in reading complex or subtle facial emotions and another's tone of voice by autistic individuals have long been identified in research (Baron-Cohen et al., 1997; Rutherford & Baron-Cohen, 2002). It is essential that a counsellor does not expect that the autistic partner can work out and spontaneously and intuitively understand what is expected of them. A very clear and direct form of communication needs to be adopted by the counsellor, especially when giving tasks, which should, if possible, be backed up with visual aids and written instructions. A counsellor should never presume that their autistic client has understood them without first checking in. Non-direct and ambiguous communication will result in feelings of confusion and being overwhelmed, and being given too much information at once and having to process multiple messages will increase stress, as shown below:

(AMP) 'Felt attacked and overwhelmed as I work better in writing and there is a lot of info to consider. I wanted to be able to take notes as I do in meetings in order to follow what is going on'.

(AFP) 'Overwhelming. Confusing. Hard to follow. Upsetting'.

It is clear from the examples above that the counselling experience was both demoralizing and disempowering and left these clients feeling lost and negative, which impacted strongly on their emotional well-being and feelings of worth.

NEGATIVE EFFECT ON EMOTIONAL WELL-BEING

Reports from the respondents were frequent and disturbing regarding the negative effect that couple counselling had had on their emotional well-being and mental health.

The aim of counselling is to benefit the clients, and to restore and build self-esteem and independence. 'Beneficence', as 'a commitment to promoting the client's well-being', is one of the five core principles stipulated in the ethical code laid down by the British Association of Counselling and Psychotherapy (BACP, 2018, p. 9). This is followed by 'non-maleficence': 'a commitment to avoiding harm to the client'.

It appears that in many cases neither of these core principles were fulfilled in the counselling. The reports that we received from the autistic partners came from many different countries across the world, as detailed in Chapter 1. The BACP ethical guidelines, which state that any harm to a client should be avoided by the counsellors at all costs, apply to any location. However, this core principle does not appear to have been adhered to, as shown in the comment below:

> (AMP) 'I thought it would change me as all the problems seemed to be my fault. But it didn't, I became more depressed, and was left feeling no one would ever be able to help me'.

Autistic individuals are already more vulnerable to depression and anxiety than the general population (Gillott & Standen, 2007). A later study by Cooper et al. (2017) found that having a positive autistic identity could protect against mental health issues, whereas having to mask or camouflage being autistic in order to feel accepted by the counsellor is likely to increase anxiety (Hull et al., 2017). It was shown in this survey that autism was often not recognized, not understood and at times totally refuted by the counsellor. Without feeling accepted and acknowledged and allowed to own their autistic identity, self-esteem will be compromised.

Results from a recent mental health survey for the National Autistic Society, working in partnership with Mind (National Autistic Society & Mind, 2021), highlighted just how vulnerable the autistic population is to mental health issues. The survey suggested that 94% of autistic adults have at some time suffered from anxiety and 83% have experienced episodes of depression. Three in ten individuals experience severe depression. In addition, the National Institute for Health and

Care Excellence (NICE, 2018) placed autistic individuals as being those at highest risk of suicide. The reports that we received from the autistic partners highlighted how, for some, the couple counselling felt damaging to their emotional and psychological well-being. This goes against the whole purpose of counselling which, regardless of the therapeutic process being employed, is there to advantage and benefit all that seek its services. This is a major fault in the system that needs to be rectified and addressed. The negative reports we received were plentiful:

(AMP) 'Expensive, psychologically damaging'.

(AMP) 'Apart from the stress of going through all that which was considerable... These sessions were an avoidable disaster. On the last session my muscles locked up the next day, presumably extreme tension'.

(AFP) 'Worsening self-worth... I can't do this'.

The two core requirements of beneficence and non-maleficence have clearly not been met in the cases reported here. Given that 14 of the 27 counsellors were made aware that one of the clients was probably autistic, and three of the counsellors professed to have knowledge of autism, it cannot be claimed that such poor and damaging outcomes were due to lack of awareness. However, only one of these 27 counsellors had received any formal training in autism. This is in direct contrast to the positive outcome group where 10 of the 15 counsellors had received some training and 12 were aware of the presence of autism. These figures further reinforce the need for counsellors to be fully trained in this area if reports like the one below are to be avoided:

(AMP) 'It led to me having a breakdown, the counsellor said I was shut down emotionally and couldn't communicate'.

RELATIONSHIP DETERIORATED (AS A CONSEQUENCE OF COUPLE COUNSELLING)

The aim of counselling is for clients to benefit from the therapeutic relationship. The present ethical guidelines for couple and marriage counsellors according to the American Association of Marriage and Family

Therapy (AAMFT) state that therapists should only continue therapy if it is 'reasonably clear that clients are benefiting from the relationship' (AAMFT, 2002–2023, 1.9 Relationship Beneficial to Client). They go on to state the importance of guiding clients to alternative 'appropriate therapeutic services if the therapist is unable or unwilling to provide professional help (AAMFT, 2002–2023, 1.10 Referrals).

These ethical codes are in place for a reason, and that is to ensure that counselling is beneficial to clients; if the counsellor feels that this is not the case, or that they are not able to provide a suitably experienced service, then the couple should be referred to a more appropriate service.

There was no mention of this happening in the reports received and some couples attended counselling for many sessions before either giving up or recognizing that it was not useful. One autistic client reported that realizing the uselessness of the counselling was the only positive they took from the sessions as it led to them finding other means of support.

The negative reports that were received from the autistic clients described how the counselling had failed both partners, by either not understanding autism or by not understanding how having an autistic partner would impact the non-autistic partner. For some autistic clients, the primary and motivating factor for attending couple counselling is the hope that the counsellor will be able to educate their partner and describe how they are not being unwilling or purposely avoiding emotional communication and spontaneous empathy. They are trying to make the relationship work, but due to difficulties in reading their partner's body language and the absence of being told explicitly what is required of them, they are not able to fulfil their partner's emotional needs. In many cases, the autistic respondents describe how their hopes for counselling were not realized, which led to a worsening of the relationship issues.

(AMP) 'Made me feel more disconnected, they [counsellors] did not understand impact of AS on non-autistic so my wife felt gaslighted'.

(AMP) 'It [counselling] served to make our difficulties seem intractable. I withdrew from my wife/my wife withdrew from me'.

Couple counselling can make the difference between a couple staying together or breaking up, and it does appear that in some cases counselling added to the pressure, the feelings of failure and the loss of hope of a future for the relationship.

> (AFP) 'Hitting a brick wall after a while / frustration. Having to go on feeling it [counselling] failed to help us'.

Sadly, if awareness and understanding of neurodiversity within counselling services is not improved, couples will continue to be let down. The respondents' poor outcomes reported in this section underline the need for counsellors to be fully trained in this area, otherwise autistic individuals, their partners and in many cases their children will continue to pay the cost, both financially and psychologically, due to a system that is sadly letting them down.

REFERENCES

American Association of Marriage and Family Therapy (AAMFT). (2002–2023). *Code of ethics*. www.aamft.org/Legal_Ethics/Code_of_Ethics.aspx

Baron-Cohen, S., Jolliffe, T., Mortimore, C., & Robertson, M. (1997). Another advanced test of Theory of Mind: Evidence from very high functioning adults with autism or Asperger syndrome. *Journal of Child Psychology and Psychiatry, 38*, 813–822.

British Association of Counselling and Psychotherapy. (2018). *BACP ethical framework for the counselling professions*. www.bacp.co.uk/media/3103/bacp-ethical-frame-work-for-the-counselling-professions-2018.pdf

Brodley, B. T. (1999). Reasons for responses expressing the therapist's frame of reference in client-centred therapy. *The Person-Centred Journal, 6*(1), 4–27.

Cassidy, S., & Rodgers, J. (2017). Understanding and prevention of suicide in autism. *Lancet Psychiatry, 4*(6), e11. https://doi.org/10.1016/S2215-0366(17)30162-1

Cooper, K., Smith, L. G. E., & Russell, A. (2017). Social identity, self-esteem, and mental health in autism. *European Journal of Social Psychology*. https://doi.org/10.1002/ejsp.2297

DeBrabander, K. M., Morrison, K. E., Jones, D. R., Faso, D. J., Chmielewski, M., & Sasson, N. J. (2019). Do first impressions of autistic adults differ between autistic and nonautistic observers? *Autism in Adulthood, 1*, 250–257. https://doi.org/10.1089/aut.2019.0018

Gillott, A., & Standen, P. J. (2007). Levels of anxiety and sources of stress in adults with autism. *Journal of Intellectual Disabilities, 11*(4), 359–370.

Hull, L., Petrides, K. V., Allison, C., Smith, P., Baron-Cohen, S., Lai, M.-C., & Mandy, W. (2017). 'Putting on my best normal': Social camouflaging in adults with autism spectrum conditions. *Journal of Autism and Developmental Disorders, 47*, 2519–2534. https://doi.org/10.1007/s10803-017-3166-5

Lai, M.-C., Lombardo, M. V., Ruigrok, A. N., Chakrabarti, B., Auyeung, B., Szatmari, P., Happé, F., & Baron-Cohen, S. (2017). Quantifying and exploring camouflaging in men and women with autism. *Autism, 21*(6), 690–702. https://doi.org/10.1177/1362361316671012

National Autistic Society & Mind. (2021). *Good practice guide*. https://s2.chorus-mk.thirdlight.com/file/24/asDKlN9as.klK7easFDsalAzTC/NAS-Good-Practice-Guide-A4.pdf

National Institute for Health and Care Excellence (NICE). (2018). *NICE guidance on preventing suicide in community and custodial settings (NG105)*. www.nice.org.uk/guidance/ng105

Nelson-Jones, R. (2009). *Introduction to counselling skills: Text and activities* (3rd ed.). Sage.

Rutherford, M., & Baron-Cohen, S. (2002). Reading the mind in the voice: A study with normal adults and adults with Asperger syndrome and high-functioning autism. *Journal of Autism and Developmental Disorders*, *32*, 189–194.

Sasson, N. J., Faso, D. J., Nugent, J., Lovell, S., Kennedy, D. P., & Grossman, R. B. (2017). Non-autistic peers are less willing to interact with those with autism based on thin slice judgments. *Scientific Reports*, *7*, 40700.

Strunz, S., Schermuck, C., Ballerstein, S., Ahlers, C., Dziobek, I., & Roepke, S. (2017). Romantic relationships and relationship satisfaction among adults with Asperger syndrome and high-functioning autism. *Journal of Clinical Psychology*, *73*(1), 113–125. https://doi.org/10.1002/jclp.22319

Tierney, S., Burns, J., & Kilbey, E. (2016). Looking behind the mask: Social coping strategies of girls on the autism spectrum. *Research in Autism Spectrum Disorders*, *23*, 73–83. https://doi.org/10.1016/j.rasd.2015.11.013

Tudor, K., & Merry, T. (2006). *Dictionary of person-centred psychology*. PCCS Books.

CHAPTER 4

The Non-Autistic Partners' Perspective on the Positives of Couple Counselling

The 184 individuals who identified as non-autistic all had partners who had received a diagnosis of Asperger's syndrome or autism. The sample consisted of 174 females, 4 males and 6 individuals who did not disclose their gender. One respondent was in a homosexual relationship.

Question 8 asked, 'What was the most useful aspect of the counselling?'

Question 10 asked, 'Do you believe the counselling had a positive effect on the relationship?' If the answer was yes, then the following Questions 11 and 12 asked, 'What were the positive effects on yourself?' and then 'your partner?'

A total of 184 individuals identified as having an autistic partner responded to the survey. As some respondents had attended couple counselling on more than one occasion, this resulted in 244 couple counselling cases; 23% reported they believed the couple counselling had led to an overall positive outcome. For the majority of these cases the counsellors had been aware of the presence of autism or had received some training in working with autism. It was also reported that in some cases the counsellor identified that the couple were neurodiverse.

For some respondents, though, the positive outcome of the counselling was that they recognized the counselling was damaging their already fragile relationship. This, for some, led them to find alternative support methods, such as joining groups and reading helpful books. Other respondents concluded that it would be better to end the relationship, as the counselling had robbed them of any remaining hope that their relationship could be 'fixed'. They felt all hope had been destroyed and reported their decision to leave as a positive. Lastly, one respondent in this group reported the only positive they felt was that the counselling resulted in a diagnosis. This is shown in the quote below:

(NAFP) 'The counselling itself was useless except for the DX [diagnosis]'.

The positive results from the couple counselling that non-autistic respondents reported can be grouped into five themes:

1. Being believed/validation

2. Increased understanding

3. Education

4. Improved communication

5. Diagnosis.

As with the autistic respondents, all these groups are strongly related and interwoven. In many cases, one group leads to another and is clearly correlated. Again, for the sake of clarification, we will explore each category individually, starting with being believed/validated.

BEING BELIEVED/VALIDATED

For the 55 non-autistic respondents who reported a positive outcome from the counselling, being believed and validated by the counsellor was the most reported benefit they felt they received.

Being believed ended the confusion they had felt, sometimes for many years, and offered the assurance and validation that they were not going crazy. The benefit for some was tremendous and restored self-concept and self-belief. Benefits to mental health and self-esteem followed, as seen in the quotes below:

(NAFP) 'I wasn't alone in seeing the chaos. It was the key to my recovery to be believed. I again trust my inner self and I don't feel a failure'.

(NAFP) 'Really believed this time and the benefits to my mental health were great'.

There were many responses regarding the positives of being validated by the counsellor and the offer of reassurance that the non-autistic partner was not going crazy.

| (NAFP) 'Validation for me, awareness of AS'.

| (NAFP) 'Validation that I am not crazy/bad/to blame'.

The importance of a client's feelings being validated by their therapist cannot be underestimated; this plays an integral role in forming a secure and trusting therapeutic alliance between client and counsellor. Validation encourages growth, learning and independence (Carson-Wong et al., 2018; Kocabas & Ustundag-Budak, 2017). The ability to offer genuine, non-judgemental validation is an essential requirement and skill for all counselling, regardless of the therapeutic process being employed.

INCREASED UNDERSTANDING

Validation and feeling understood are very close companions, and it is probably impossible to feel understood without feeling validated and vice versa.

Within Maxine's work as a couple counsellor, she has heard endless accounts of feelings of utter confusion when awareness of autism is lacking. The majority of the non-autistic partners she has worked with love their partners but declare they have no understanding of their partner's behaviour and responses towards them and their relationship. Many non-autistic partners, especially when they are female in the relationship, express that their gut feeling tells them their partner's behaviour and lack of emotional response is not intentional or deliberate.

Some non-autistic partners will have spent years trying to figure out why their partner behaves in such a way, why they don't feel their partner understands them or is even aware of the sadness and loneliness they feel. They may have spent years exploring their partner's childhood experiences and upbringing, searching for an explanation for the differences in their partner's emotional responses and perceived aloofness. The majority will come to counselling to find answers to often desperate questions. They need someone else to observe and witness the confusion they are experiencing and to explain to them why they feel so lonely and often unloved by their partner, as seen in the quote below:

(NAFP) 'It [counselling] let me know I was not to blame for wanting to be more loved and understood'.

Understanding that all individuals express love differently and that different does not mean less is key to relationship satisfaction. Not having any knowledge about how being autistic can affect how love is expressed can leave the non-autistic partner feeling unloved, because they don't know how to recognize love being displayed in a non-traditional way. This is because the non-autistic partner will be looking for love to be expressed in a form and language they understand. The autistic partner's love language may well be different to their non-autistic partner's. It may be that love is less likely to be expressed through meaningful words but rather through actions, such as working hard, being a provider or simply making their partner a cup of tea. For example, as reported by the female non-autistic partner below, a positive she received from the counselling was:

(NAFP) 'Understood that we thought in totally different ways'.

Understanding the WHY is empowering and offers control over what may have felt like a powerless situation. Lack of understanding can produce fear, confusion and uncertainty, and strip an individual of their feelings of confidence, trust and control. The knowledge that the counsellor understands both partners and can help both to understand each other is one of the keys to good counselling.

For a partner to feel that they are understood on a deeper level is productive and beneficial to the well-being and strength of the couple's relationship.

For an autistic individual, their acquired knowledge of their partner can be quite strong; however, their subjective understanding of their partner, unless things are clearly explained, can be misled by misunderstandings. This is not intentional, but unless the non-autistic partner can explain clearly how they feel, their feelings are likely to be overlooked or misread by their autistic partner.

Without the knowledge that their partner is autistic, the non-autistic partner is likely to interpret the autistic partner's perceived lack of understanding as not caring enough or not being concerned about them. The counsellor's ability to show the non-autistic partner that they understand how they feel, and to explain how these misunderstandings are more likely due to the couple being unaware they belong in a neu-rodiverse relationship, is critical in building trust and confidence in the counselling process. Without this trust in the counsellor, it will be difficult or impossible for the non-autistic partner to make any progress and bring into effect appropriate changes to how they respond to and perceive their autistic partner. This is shown in the following positive examples:

> (NAFP) 'I am less confused and frustrated by his behaviour, I under-stand why he behaves the way he does'.

Having an understanding of autism will allow for the learning of new skills to improve the daily running of the relationship, and will also highlight the need for the non-autistic partner to take the responsibility of finding alternative ways to get their needs met.

> (NAFP) 'Becoming more self-reliant and understanding that I cannot rely heavily on him'.

> (NAFP) 'Counsellor understanding his symptoms and having prac-tical solutions'.

EDUCATION

During the many years that we have worked with neurodiverse couples, we have found that often, our primary role in the counselling room has been that of educator. Autism is not just a word. It is a complex condi-tion that will affect every individual differently. Autism does not change individuality, personality, childhood experiences, beliefs or opinions. Every person who is autistic will be unique. This, we believe, is the basic foundation on which all learning should take place. Every autistic individual is unique and should be treated accordingly.

The core traits of autism, however, are not unique, and the traits will be the same for every autistic person, although the severity of each trait and the direction it takes will be different for everyone. To make it even more complex, the severity of the traits is not static, and they will change according to the individual's stress level and the situation and context they find themselves in.

For example, many of the female non-autistic partners Maxine has worked with describe their confusion over why their autistic partner can manage at work, sometimes under great pressure, hold meetings and have conversations with colleagues, and yet as soon as they arrive home and are with the family, they become stressed, uncommunicative and uninvolved.

The first thing to do in this situation is to ask what the autistic partner does as a job, and to discover they may be, for example, a dentist or an accountant. Some autistic individuals may have found employment within an area that is also their special interest. In other words, it is a place where they are the expert and are firmly within their comfort zone. No one in the workplace is likely to be seeking out conversations regarding emotional feelings or that require mind and body reading. Having said that, we have encountered autistic individuals who do work within the caring professions and are able to do this proficiently, once it is understood clearly what is required of them.

Within the family environment, the expectations are very different; there will be conversations that are emotional, and situations that will require reading body language. The family environment can be very unpredictable, and spontaneous reactions are often expected. The autistic partner may feel out of their comfort zone or will be feeling totally depleted and exhausted from the demands they have managed in their working day. Ideally, this is when the autistic individual should be allowed time to re-energize and make the transition from working life to family life.

A counsellor who understands autism will understand why this occurs and will be able to explain to the non-autistic partner the reasons why and educate them on what they can do to improve the situation for both them and their autistic partner.

Having an understanding of autism and how it affects both the individual and the relationship will promote learning and encourage change and adjustment. The examples given by the non-autistic partners below show quite clearly how learning was beneficial to both them and their partner:

(NAFP) 'Learnt more about relating to partner in useful ways'.

(NAFP) 'Learning to understand my husband's way of thinking (or not) about me and our marriage'.

In intimate relationships, the main focus of learning will be on making improvements in the communication that takes place between the couple. This takes us to the next positive outcome that the non-autistic partners reported had been achieved from the couple counselling.

IMPROVED COMMUNICATION

Communication is the primary area of concern and dissatisfaction highlighted by couples when one partner is autistic. By the time a couple find their way into the counselling room, they are likely to have experienced years of communication breakdown, have a whole catalogue of past misunderstandings and, due to the difficulties in communication, have an accumulation of unresolved issues.

When a counsellor is working with a neurodiverse couple, they can find themselves working as a translator or interpreter, as both partners will often appear to be talking in totally different languages. The communication of the autistic partner can be quite logical and to the point, whereas the language of the non-autistic partner may be less direct and involve more emotional language. The two will struggle to understand each other and frequently misinterpret the true intent behind the other's communication. It is likely, due to difficulties in mind and body reading, that the autistic partner will be hearing most of what their partner communicates as criticism; this will, in turn, provoke a very defensive and self-protective reaction.

The long-term effect of constant misunderstandings will be a complete breakdown in communication. The counsellor's role will be to offer skills and strategies to improve communication. This will be one of the primary steps towards rebuilding trust within the couple relationship. To restore trust in communication it is essential that the couple feel it is safe to do so. If the therapeutic alliance between the couple and counsellor is weak, this will not be achieved. Both in the relationship have to feel safe and trust in the counsellor's ability to only set them tasks and teach them skills that are within their ability. A counsellor who understands neurodiversity and has personal experience or training in this area should have the acquired sensitivity to formulate and devise a plan with the couple that works for both of them. Without this precursor in place, it is likely that anything that follows will fail. From the positive report below from a non-autistic partner, we can see that this was achieved:

(NAFP) 'Vastly improved connection and communication. Much reduced Cassandra complex [see Chapter 10]'.

Once a trusting therapeutic alliance is in place and a way forward has been agreed with the couple, the counsellor can go on to teach the couple alternative and more constructive ways to communicate. This is shown in the quotes below:

(NAFP) 'She [counsellor] was able to give us some good communication tools'.

(NAFP) 'Counsellor gave us communication strategies that were helpful'.

Sometimes it will feel to both partners that they have been struggling for years to try to make things work and adjust their lifestyle and habits. By the time they arrive in the counselling room, they are both probably already suffering from relationship fatigue.

Consequently, it can come as a pleasant surprise and relief to learn that the majority of adjustments and skills to be learnt can be quite simple and require little effort. The majority of skills required can be easily learnt by both counsellor and couple. We will be discussing these skills more in Chapter 20.

Communication is a two-way process; not only do the couple need to learn ways to send accurate messages to their partner, they also need to learn to listen to what their partner is saying. It is not uncommon for non-autistic partners to feel unheard and that their autistic partner is not interested in what they have to say. There are various reasons for this. For some, it is because their autistic partner becomes quickly defensive and reacts by either talking over them or simply shutting down and not listening. Another common cause is distraction caused by poor timing of communication, such as having discussions while the television is turned on. A further reason is that autistic individuals may have difficulty with attentive listening, such that they may be listening but not looking at their conversation partner or expressing appropriate non-verbal communication such as nodding or appropriate facial and gestural expression.

The counselling room can be an ideal place to practice communication skills, as all distractions and sensory triggers are removed and mobiles are turned off (see Chapter 9). This will enable both partners to focus entirely on each other and what is being said. The counselling room should be the ideal place for learning and enable the couple to develop skills they can take home to practice in their own environment. As reported by one non-autistic woman below:

(NAFP) 'Learning to take turns listening to each other'.

Another aspect of communication that was reported as a positive outcome from the counselling sessions was learning how each expressed their love. All individuals will express their love for their partner differently, and individuals will look to receive love back in the same way they give it. This is perfectly natural and our unique love language is probably learnt at an early age from our parents.

Dr Gary Chapman discusses this in detail in his bestselling book *The Five Love Languages* (1992). Chapman argues that how we express our love can be narrowed down into five languages, and it is important for those in a couple to recognize what their languages are and, equally important, what their partner's are. For example, if the non-autistic partner's primary love language is words of affirmation, and this is how they look to their partner to show their love back, I am afraid they may be disappointed, as words are less likely to be the preferred way for an autistic partner to show their love. The autistic partner is more likely to be comfortable showing their love by acts of service, such as doing jobs and providing for their family. Words of affirmation can be difficult for an autistic partner, sometimes due to not intuitively knowing what to say and fear of saying the wrong thing or not coming across as genuine. The logical and practical mind of an autistic partner, especially if the partner is male, will find 'doing' rather than 'saying' both safer and more meaningful. Understanding this can for the non-autistic partner prove both fruitful and confidence building.

All four positives reported by the 55 non-autistic respondents in the survey that we've discussed so far are very closely linked, and it is not possible to say which came first in the counselling process, as all are dependent on the other. What can be said from these positive reports is how much of the progress the couple experienced was dependent on the counsellor being aware of autism within an intimate relationship. The fifth positive reported from couple counselling was that it resulted in a diagnostic assessment for autism.

DIAGNOSIS

Nine of the non-autistic respondents reported that due to the expertise of the counsellor, it was recognized that their partner was autistic. Becoming aware that autism is present can open many doors and choices to a couple that were not available before. Not all the respondents discovered autism directly from the counsellor; for some it was brought into the couple's awareness indirectly through the couple counselling sessions, as seen below:

> (NAFP) 'The DX came indirectly from counselling has changed my expectations and understanding so our relationship is more viable'.

Nine, though, did come directly from the counsellor and resulted in many positive changes in the relationship. When it comes to neurodiversity, ignorance is not bliss; this will inevitably result in misunderstandings, failed expectations and, in the worst case scenario, separation and divorce, which often could have been avoided. Knowledge is empowering and motivational, and essential if the counselling is going to feel safe and appropriate for the couple, as seen in the quotes below:

> (NAFP) 'The DX allowed him to understand himself, the DX helped me to show him I love him in a way he could understand. Once we understood we could start to recover'.

Unfortunately for many of the non-autistic respondents the results from the couple counselling were negative rather than positive, and this brings us onto our next chapter, which will explore the negative experiences of the non-autistic respondents.

REFERENCES

Carson-Wong, A., Hughes, C. D., & Rizvi, S. L. (2018). The effect of therapist use of validation strategies on change in client emotion in individual DBT treatment sessions. *Personality Disorders: Theory, Research, and Treatment*, 9(2), 165–171. https://doi.org/10.1037/per0000229

Chapman, G. (1992). *The five love languages*. Northfield Publishing.

Kocabas, E., & Ustundag-Budak, M. (2017). Validation skills in counselling and psychotherapy. *International Journal of Scientific Study*, 5(8), 319–322.

CHAPTER 5

The Non-Autistic Partners' Perspective on the Negatives of Couple Counselling

Question 9 asked, 'What was the least useful aspect of the counselling?'

Question 13 asked 'Do you believe the counselling had a negative effect on the relationship? If the answer was yes then Questions 14 and 15 asked 'If yes, what were the negative effects on yourself?' and then 'your partner?'

Over 77% (189) of respondents reported they believed the couple counselling had led to some negative outcomes and over half of these reported an overall negative outcome.

The majority of the counsellors involved in the negative outcomes were known to have not had any training in working with autism, and in two cases counsellors claimed to have knowledge of autism but this was disputed by the couple.

The negative results that respondents reported experiencing fit into four themes:

- Lack of understanding and support

- Not being believed/validated

- Negative effect on emotional well-being

- Relationship deteriorated due to the counselling.

As with the autistic respondents, all these themes are strongly related and interwoven. In many cases, one theme leads to another, and they are clearly linked. Again, for the sake of clarity, we will explore each theme individually, starting with a lack of understanding by the counsellor.

LACK OF UNDERSTANDING AND SUPPORT

Many of the responses received from the non-autistic respondents reported that autism was not understood by the counsellor and, as a consequence, the non-autistic partner was not understood either. Living with an autistic partner means living with a partner who thinks differently and processes information differently. This difference is often very subtle and can be, for the non-autistic partner, extremely difficult to put into words and describe.

What makes it even more difficult to describe is that the non-autistic partner is often aware that a difference exists but does not know the cause and cannot make sense of why the same misunderstandings keep repeating themselves. It is rarely the intention of the autistic partner to ignore or not respond appropriately to their partner's emotional needs. This apparent lack of spontaneous emotional reciprocity is due to the fact that the autistic partner is often totally unaware that their partner has needs that are not being fulfilled. This is because these needs are rarely conveyed in words, but rather are communicated non-verbally via facial expressions and body language.

Being autistic can restrict a person's ability to spontaneously read another's thoughts and intentions accurately (Attwood, 2006, p. 114). If no verbal direction and explanation is offered to the autistic partner, it is unlikely they will be fully aware a message is being sent or they will not interpret the message correctly. For example, due to difficulties interpreting voice tone and emphasis, a message that was intended to be helpful could easily be heard as negative or a criticism.

It might be easier to understand if, rather than using the word autistic, the example of one partner being hard of hearing was used. Being hard of hearing can cause someone to only pick up on specific tones, so sometimes only part of a message is heard. Now imagine that this person was unaware they were hard of hearing, as was their partner. This would create a catalogue of misunderstandings in the relationship for both, but especially the hearing (non-autistic) partner. If no response was given to their message, they would be left feeling either ignored or uncared for. If they believed their partner had heard their message and then couldn't recall it accurately, they would be left feeling irrelevant. Finally, if their message was misinterpreted as negative or critical when they meant well, they would be left feeling very misunderstood. If the couple do not discover that their partner is hard of hearing and this pattern continues, it will start to feel personal and negative feelings will grow. The only way this can be changed is to discover why these miscommunications have occurred and set up strategies and ways of coping to improve how they converse.

This is one of the reasons why it is so important that autism is recognized and accepted. Otherwise, the non-autistic partner will continue to have expectations that their autistic partner cannot always meet. Difficulties in reading non-verbal expressions and body language will cause misunderstandings and a lack of spontaneous emotional reciprocity in the relationship if one partner is autistic. However, if the non-autistic partner is not aware they are in a neurodiverse relationship, or they do not understand the consequences that being autistic can have, they will have spent sometimes years trying to describe to friends and family how the relationship is making them feel lonely and uncared for. For many, they will not have been understood by friends and family, and the difficulties they are trying to describe will not have been acknowledged or recognized.

The non-autistic partner will enter couple counselling with a strong hope that a professional couple counsellor will understand their feelings. They will have expectations that the counsellor will be able to empathize with their situation and how they feel. However, for the majority of non-autistic respondents in our survey, this clearly did not happen. Many described being misunderstood because the counsellor had no understanding of autism or neurodiverse relationships. The non-autistic women in a study in Japan also reported feeling they and their relationship situation was not understood by family, friends or counsellors (Deguchi & Asakura, 2018).

(NAFP) 'Counsellor didn't understand, know about AS'.

(NAFP) 'She [counsellor] did not understand my husband and she did not understand my experience of him'.

Once again, as also described by the autistic respondents in this survey, inappropriate tasks and activities were given that were unachievable and impossible to maintain for the autistic partner. This had, for many, a devastating and demoralizing effect on the autistic partner and reinforced feelings of failure that were described by many of the autistic respondents in this study.

In couple counselling, much importance and relevance is placed upon the counsellor's responsibility to ensure that the couple counselling provided does not disadvantage either partner and is not biased towards one client over another. To recommend and give tasks and strategies that are inappropriate for one within the couple relationship would cause an imbalance of power, and both partners would consequently suffer and be left with feelings of hopelessness and failure.

(NAFP) 'Therapist did not understand AS and suggested impossible things for my husband'.

(NAFP) 'Kept being asked to do things he [husband] wasn't capable of'.

The above statements reinforce the importance of a counsellor understanding the couple they are counselling. Only with this understanding and awareness will the counsellor be able to work in an appropriate and beneficial way to address the couple's relationship. Without an understanding of autism and the dynamics and limitations of being in a neurodiverse relationship, the counsellor will be counselling from a non-autistic perspective, and expectations will be placed on the couple that are unrealistic and unachievable. In many cases, neither the couple nor the counsellor was aware of the presence of autism in the relationship. Having said that, 50% of this group reporting negative outcomes did make the counsellor aware of their partner's autism, and still the counselling and tasks given were inappropriate. For the couple counselling to benefit both partners, the counsellor needs to have a thorough knowledge of what it means to be autistic and equally what it means for a non-autistic individual to live with an autistic partner. The British Association of Counselling and Psychotherapy (2018, p. 14) is very clear in stating the importance of a counsellor working to a professional standard, as seen in the statement below:

Working to professional standards 13. We must be competent to deliver the services being offered to at least fundamental professional standards or better. When we consider satisfying professional standards requires consulting others with relevant expertise, seeking second opinions, or making referrals.

This statement is very clear in its directive and goes on to recommend how working to professional standards might be achieved in the following statements, shown below:

14. We will keep skills and knowledge up to date by:

    a. reading professional journals, books and/or reliable electronic resources

    b. keeping ourselves informed of any relevant research and evidence-based guidance

    c. discussions with colleagues working with similar issues

    d. reviewing our knowledge and skills in supervision or discussion with experienced practitioners

    e. regular continuing professional development to update knowledge and skills.

It is the duty of a counsellor to ensure that they are competent and experienced enough to be working with the clients they counsel. If in doubt, they should refer their clients to a professional who has the relevant skills. If the clients choose to stay with their present counsellor or there is no one to refer them to, then the counsellor needs to take all measures available to them to bring their knowledge up to date. If the counsellor does not take action and attempts to provide their clients counselling with the knowledge they already have, couples will continue to be let down and for some, psychologically damaged by the counselling experience.

The statement below given by a non-autistic partner shows that, in their case, this necessary requirement was not met:

(NAFP) 'I felt betrayed. This time by a professional'.

Many respondents were left with feelings of hopelessness and in a far worse place than when they started the counselling process. They described how their feelings of loneliness and isolation were exacerbated due to the lack of understanding from the counsellor.

(NAFP) 'I gave up hope of finding a counsellor who would understand'.

(NAFP) 'I felt no one really had the skills to help so I felt even more isolated and misunderstood'.

Others were left feeling as though they were invisible and unacknowledged, which leads us to our next closely related theme of not feeling believed or validated.

NOT BEING BELIEVED/VALIDATED

The majority of the couples that we have encountered over the years had no awareness that one partner was autistic when they first met. Many couples had been together for decades before the possibility was discovered that autism could be the cause for the confusion and discontent in their relationship.

It is only in the past ten years that awareness of autism among adults has become more widespread. In 1996, the National Autistic Society (NAS) conducted a large survey into the experiences and attitudes of the general public towards autism (NAS, 1996). A section of this survey interviewed 979 people from all regions of Great Britain to discover how many had heard of Asperger's syndrome (now referred to as autism). The survey found that only 4% of the participants reported having heard of Asperger's syndrome. The NAS then asked how many participants had heard of Stirling syndrome, to which a total of 3% claimed they had. Considering that Stirling syndrome is a fictional condition the findings of this survey show clearly how few members of the general public had any knowledge of the existence of Asperger's syndrome.

This survey was conducted 27 years ago; in our present survey, the average length of relationship for the couples was 21 years. So it is doubtful that many of our respondents would have any knowledge of autism, especially as it used to be considered primarily a childhood disorder.

For those non-autistic partners who were unaware that their partner was autistic, it is quite probable that the early expectations for the relationship would have been very high and based entirely on unachievable hopes and aspirations. In the initial stages of the relationship, it is likely that the autistic partner would have been making a great deal of effort in trying to form a secure connection with the non-autistic partner of their choice. Masking would be in full swing to fulfil the strong desire by the autistic partner to be liked and attractive to their prospective partner. This may have taken various forms, from buying expensive gifts to being totally attentive to the other's needs.

Such attentive behaviour can prove strongly appealing to non-autistic partners, who often described how special and highly desirable they felt during this initial period of the relationship. Feeling totally enamoured by so much attention, the courtship can soon develop into something much deeper, and it is seldom long before marriage or moving in together takes place.

This is often the point that everything changes, as now the secure attachment has been made, the autistic partner can step back and relax into a more comfortable, familiar lifestyle, which unfortunately often does not take into account their new partner. This process may happen over a period of time, and initially the non-autistic partner will be trying to find explanations for the change in attitude and behaviour. They may look for reasons and excuses for the autistic partner's lack of emotional response. For example, they may blame their partner's emotional absence on their workload or upbringing. In an attempt to get their needs met and restore the equilibrium in the relationship, some non-autistic partners may try harder to be more accommodating of their partner's needs by not being too emotionally demanding. It is at this time that a sense of loneliness in the relationship may begin to creep in for the non-autistic partner.

The next stage of the relationship can, for some, see the arrival of children, and this will totally change the focus of the relationship. If the non-autistic partner is the primary carer, the new arrivals will quickly become their main focus of care and attention. Whilst this may offer a sense of belonging and purpose, it can soon become apparent to the non-autistic partner that they are managing all the childcare alone and the whole responsibility for the family's welfare appears to be placed solely on their shoulders.

Meanwhile, the autistic partner may be totally unaware that anything is amiss, believing that the role they have taken, which is often one of provider, is sufficient. When looking at relationship satisfaction in neurodivergent couples, autistic partners often report higher satisfaction than their non-autistic partners (Strunz et al., 2017). Misguided assumptions might be made by the autistic partner, and they are likely to believe that the non-autistic partner is content with the relationship and satisfied with the level of effort and contribution they are putting into their family.

It can come as a great surprise to the autistic partner when they are informed that their partner is not happy, and they are likely to struggle to understand why the non-autistic partner appears to be critical and complaining. The autistic partner may be very shocked to discover that their partner is not content and react defensively to what they may describe as a personal attack by the non-autistic partner. There could be a total denial of the accusation, putting doubt in the non-autistic partner's mind, often leaving them confused and questioning whether they are being unreasonable and ungrateful. Doubts will creep in, slowly engulfing self-esteem and sense of self. Before seeking counselling services, the non-autistic partner may have tried talking to family and friends and might have even approached their GP. It is likely that they will have found themselves not being believed, as on the outside there often do not appear to be any problems or issues in the relationship.

The relationship can now find itself spiralling downwards, and it is often, at this time, that the non-autistic partner arranges for them both to attend couple counselling. The hope for the non-autistic partner is that they will be believed by the counsellor, and the counsellor will understand how they feel. Unfortunately, for many in this survey, their hopes went unfulfilled, and their feelings of loneliness and self-doubt increased.

Not being believed and validated by the counsellor made up a high proportion of the negative experiences reported by the non-autistic respondents who attended couple counselling.

(NAFP) 'I was disbelieved about the difficulties in our relationship'.

(NAFP) 'Made me more frustrated, disbelieved and lonely'.

Feelings of loneliness have been described by many non-autistic partners we have worked with. Loneliness has been found to be a key contributor to the struggles experienced by non-autistic women in neurodiverse relationships (Deguchi & Asakura, 2018). In their study, conducted in Japan, Deguchi and Asakura give an example of a non-autistic wife who described that although living with her husband she felt they were divided by a glass partition, and that she was unable to get her feelings through to him. She and others described in the study a sense of loneliness.

If an individual does not feel their reality is understood, believed and validated this will create a loss of self-esteem and nurture feelings of self-doubt, including of one's sanity. Emotional focused therapy cites validation as a key intervention in couple therapy (Johnson, 2007). Johnson argues that validation removes fears of judgement and self-criticism. Validation also supplies the reassurance of safety and trust in the therapeutic alliance that a client needs to explore their feelings and perceptions further.

Without validation of a client's reality from a counsellor it would not be possible for the therapeutic relationship to grow and for any positive outcome to be achieved. Without validation of one's reality then self-doubt will increase, as shown in the quotes below:

(NAFP) 'I don't feel believed or validated enough'.

(NAFP) 'At times it increased the hopelessness, alienation and isolation and sometimes invalidation'.

It is also essential in couple therapy that the experience of both clients in the relationship, regardless of whether they are expressing different perspectives, should be validated equally by the counsellor. This parallel validation is essential to avoid any bias towards one client. The non-autistic respondents reported on many occasions that they believed the counsellor was negatively biased against them, and this consequently had a damaging effect on their relationship and left them feeling responsible for the difficulties they were both experiencing.

(NAFP) 'Not being believed and also being blamed'.

(NAFP) 'Lowered self-esteem, blamed and suicidal'.

This does bring into question why, in so many instances, it was reported by both the autistic and the non-autistic respondent that they believed the counsellor favoured the autistic partner over the non-autistic partner. Research has found that it is more likely to be the non-autistic partner who is in distress and seeking support (Smith et al., 2020), while autistic partners often report higher relationship satisfaction rates (Strunz et al., 2017). It is therefore likely that both partners will be entering the counselling services with a different agenda and a different set of needs.

With the many couples we have worked with, particularly when the autistic partner is male and the non-autistic partner is either female or a male in a homosexual relationship, it is the non-autistic partner that will often present in the counselling room as emotional, frustrated and sometimes angry. This will be in direct contrast to the autistic partner who, often due to masking, will appear calm, reserved and polite and often appear totally unaware of why they are there. Their main focus will be to learn how to make their partner happy and they will often express this to the counsellor.

If the counsellor has not received any training in working with neurodiversity, their perceptions and observations could affect how they react to each partner and create an impression of being seemingly biased. The counsellor will find themselves drawn into an unrealistic and false image of the relationship. Unfortunately, this bias and lack of validation for non-autistic clients will continue if training and awareness remain neglected.

Being believed and validated reinforces a sense of self and avoids feelings of anxiety and self-doubt. If this is not offered, it is likely to have a strong impact on the client's emotional well-being, as seen in the statement below, and the following section:

> (NAFP) 'I was disbelieved about the difficulties in our relationship. It made me feel even more worthless and disbelieved. Suicidal'.

NEGATIVE EFFECT ON EMOTIONAL WELL-BEING

Negative reports of the damaging effect that couple counselling had on the non-autistic respondent and their autistic partner were plentiful and very concerning.

> (NAFP) 'Incredibly damaging to self-esteem'.

> (NAFP) 'Increased stress and a sense of hopelessness'.

Reports of doubting one's sanity are very common in the non-autistic partner, especially when there is no awareness of the presence of autism and its effects. The term Cassandra syndrome (or Cassandra phenomenon, among other terms) has been around for over 20 years and has been used to describe the effect of living in a neurodiverse relationship on the non-autistic partner (see Chapter 10). The Cassandra effect is strongest when neither partner is aware that they are in a neurodiverse relationship. Being made aware of the neurological difference between them can greatly lessen the Cassandra effect, especially if both partners can develop an understanding and acceptance of what this means. Lefebvre and Hunsley (1994) found in their case study that when a couple were made aware that the difficulties in their relationship were caused by a neurological difference, such as autism, rather than the behaviour of the partners, the relationship improved. Awareness and acceptance are essential to achieving and maintain a healthy relationship. This adds to why it is so important for a therapist to be trained to recognize, understand and be able to help and support a neurodiverse couple in this way. If this is lacking in couple counselling, then the effects of Cassandra syndrome will increase, and positive outcomes are unlikely to be achieved.

Without awareness and understanding many non-autistic partners can over time begin to doubt their own opinions and self, questioning their own sanity as they try to make sense of why communication and intimacy with their partner is so difficult to achieve. Validation of not being 'crazy' was one of the key positives received by those non-autistic partners who had a good experience, as described in Chapter 4. In the negative reports, however, feeling crazy and doubting one's sanity were reinforced by the counselling, as shown in the statements below:

(NAFP) 'I felt more crazy'.

(NAFP) 'I felt invalidated...and I'm left feeling Cassandra syndrome'.

Another effect of living in a neurodiverse relationship for the non-autistic partner is that they may begin, over a period of time, to repress their emotions (Deguchi & Asakura, 2018). This can happen slowly and begins when the non-autistic partner realizes that being emotional does not benefit them in any way and can have an adverse effect on their partner. Due to the autistic partner's difficulties interpreting body language and vocal tone, the non-autistic partner's emotions will frequently be seen as negative. Consequently, feelings of sadness, feeling down or having a bad day will frequently be interpreted by the autistic partner as being angry at them. Believing their partner is angry at them will often cause one of three reactions in the autistic partner: fight, flight or freeze. The fight reaction could cause a defensive or angry response, as they may believe they are under attack; flight means retreating to another room or leaving the house altogether; freeze could be a total shutdown, manifesting as refusing to respond or communicate, which could last for days or more. Consequently, over time, the non-autistic partner will try to repress their feelings, as showing them will not be productive. This way, they will avoid upsetting their partner or being made to feel bad about themselves.

Suppressing emotions has been found to be associated with the symptoms of depression (Feldman et al., 2008), particularly the suppression of feelings of anger. Displays of anger, even healthy anger, achieve very little in neurodiverse relationships. For many of the autistic adults we have worked with there is a profound fear of confrontation, and they will do whatever is in their power to avoid this. Regardless of whether the anger is appropriate to the situation and expressed in a healthy way, this is needed to clear the air to resolve disagreements. Difficulties over the non-autistic partners' expression of feelings may be increased as they are likely to find all their feelings being misinterpreted by their autistic partner as being angry. This is due to the difficulty the autistic partner may have in reading their partner's emotions accurately and due to their own feelings of low self-esteem; this leads them to assume that what is being said is negative when the intention was supportive or positive.

The non-autistic partner will quickly learn that if anything is to be achieved in the relationship, they will have to supress any feelings of anger. Unfortunately, a consequence of this can be the onset of depression, and if not checked, this can become a major concern for the non-autistic partner. Feelings could be further suppressed over time as the non-autistic partner will not be able to openly discuss how they feel with their autistic partner for fear of provoking a negative reaction. This could ultimately increase depressive symptoms. A study by Arad et al. (2022) found significantly higher levels of depression (47%) in non-autistic respondents in a neurodiverse relationship compared to 13% in the control group.

(NAMP) 'Feeling let down and depressed'.

(NAFP) 'Increase in despair and desperation. Made me feel worse, depressed'.

Meanwhile the autistic partner will be aware that something is wrong but not know what. Some will blame themselves for the state their partner is in:

63

(NAFP) 'He became frustrated with himself when he failed to meet my expectation. He shut down for months at a time. It was awful'.

Other autistic partners will equally feel disillusioned by the counselling, especially when it fails to result in any benefit to either.

(NAFP) 'My husband thought it was a waste of time... I was deeply depressed and feeling suicidal'.

If the non-autistic partner finds themselves not understood or their experience not validated by their counsellor, it is likely these constrained, repressed emotions will release themselves in the counselling room and years of suppressed anger and frustration might come to the forefront. The non-autistic partner will be expressing all the anger for both of them; this could give the impression that the autistic partner is the victim in the relationship. The counsellor will not be observing an accurate picture of the internal workings and dynamics of the relationship and could develop a biased view against the non-autistic partner, hence reinforcing their feelings of not being believed or understood. This could damage both partners' self-esteem and reinforce feelings of being blamed and self-doubt, as seen in the reports below.

(NAFP) 'Incredibly damaging to self-esteem'.

(NAFP) 'Lowered self-esteem, blamed and suicidal'.

Accounts of non-autistic partners feeling suicidal as a result of the counselling were of a very similar nature to those of the autistic partners in Chapter 3. The countless negative reports received in this survey were disturbing, and without doubt highlighted the need for couple counsellors to be trained in working with neurodiverse relationships. Without appropriate training, couple counselling will continue to prove both traumatic and damaging to neurodiverse couples and the negative experiences described by the couples in this survey will continue to be lived out in the counselling room.

(NAFP) 'Useless and utterly destructive to my mental health and marriage'.

(NAMP) 'A very bad experience for both of us. I now feel stressed and feel we have exhausted our options. I would say we are both worse off mentally as a result of trying to get help'.

RELATIONSHIP DETERIORATED DUE TO THE COUNSELLING

Many reports from non-autistic respondents stated that they believed their relationships were in a worse state at the end of the counselling than when they first attended. These reports were received from both male and female respondents, all living with an autistic partner.

The blame for the deterioration and damage to the relationship was placed on the counselling received rather than any deterioration or damage caused by the couple themselves. The reasons given for this fall into three groups. The first group was due to the feelings of hopelessness that the counselling provoked and reinforced.

(NAFP) 'Increased hopelessness and hurt, failure, inflamed a volatile situation'.

The second group was caused by the counsellor not recognizing autism or having no understanding of its impact in a neurodiverse relationship.

(NAFP) 'He no longer admits he has any kind of condition...an absolute disaster for our family'.

The third group was where autism was recognized but not understood, and was handled inappropriately with unsuitable exercises and advice given.

(NAFP) 'We weren't given specific changes or activities or strategies to employ or rehearse'.

Although these groups are all different, they all originate from the same cause: the lack of knowledge, expertise and training of the counsellor when working with neurodiverse couples.

Training in counselling neurodiverse relationships is both scarce and expensive, but is available in some locations or online. However, undertaking this training is voluntary and down to the individual counsellor to pursue, find the time for and pay for themselves. This training, for many counsellors, may not feel necessary or relevant enough if they do not intend to specialize in this area. However, as the number of neurodiverse couples seeking relationship counselling is increasing, it is inevitable that more counsellors will find themselves face to face or working online with a neurodiverse couple who may or may not be aware that one or both are autistic. This couple will be coming to counselling with the hope that a professional will help them make sense of why they are struggling to make their relationship work. Sometimes coming to couple counselling is the last chance for the relationship to be restored.

Couples will be looking to the counsellor to be understanding, to increase their awareness and to educate them on the best possible way of improving their relationship. At present, too many couples are being let down by the counselling they receive, and too many counsellors are not getting the training they require.

(NAFP) 'It brought a lot of negative emotion to the surface and made life more difficult for some time afterwards'.

(NAFP) 'Counselling made every aspect worse. His anxiety increased, and he was abusive to me'.

The statements above are disturbing and not only highlight how the counselling worsened the state of the relationships; it also put some clients at risk, not just by increasing mental health issues, but also by leaving some feeling under threat from their partner. This was squarely due to the counselling these couples received, so it is unlikely that they will be motivated to repeat the process, leaving the couple with all doors to support firmly closed and feeling very let down by the counselling service they received.

REFERENCES

Arad, P., Shechtman, Z., & Attwood, T. (2022). Physical and mental well-being of women in neurodiverse relationships: A comparative study. *Journal of Psychology and Psychotherapy*, *12*(1), 1000420.

Attwood, T. (2006). *The complete guide to Asperger's syndrome*. Jessica Kingsley Publishers.

British Association of Counselling and Psychotherapy. (2018). *BACP ethical framework for the counselling professions*. www.bacp.co.uk/media/3103/bacp-ethical-framework-for-the-counselling-professions-2018.pdf

Deguchi, N., & Asakura, T. (2018). Qualitative study of wives of husbands with autism spectrum disorder: Subjective experience of wives from marriage to marital crisis. *Psychology*, *9*, 14–33. https://doi.org/10.4236/psych.2018.91002

Feldman, G. C., Joormann, J., & Johnson, S. L. (2008). Responses to positive affect: A self-report measure of rumination and dampening. *Cognitive Therapy and Research, 32*(4), 507–525. https://doi.org/10.1007/s10608-006-9083-0

Johnson, S. M. (2007). The contribution of emotionally focused couples therapy. *Journal of Contemporary Psychotherapy, 37*, 47–52. https://doi.org/10.1007/s10879-006-9034-9

Lefebvre, M., & Hunsley, J. (1994). Couple's accounts of the effects of individual psychotherapy. *Psychotherapy: Theory, Research, Practice, Training, 31*(1), 183–189. https://doi.org/10.1037/0033-3204.31.1.183

National Autistic Society (NAS). (1996). *Beyond Rain Man.* NAS.

Smith, R., Netto, J., Gribble, N., & Falkmer, M. (2020). 'At the end of the day, it's love': An exploration of relationships in neurodiverse couples. *Journal of Autism and Developmental Disorders, 51*(9), 3311–3321. https://doi.org/10.1007/s10803-020-04790-z

Strunz, S., Schermuck, C., Ballerstein, S., Ahlers, C., Dziobek, I., & Roepke, S. (2017). Romantic relationships and relationship satisfaction among adults with Asperger syndrome and high-functioning autism. *Journal of Clinical Psychology, 73*(1), 113–125. https://doi.org/10.1002/jclp.22319

CHAPTER 6

How Could Current Relationship Counselling Be Improved When a Partner Has Autistic Characteristics?

Respondents in the survey were asked whether they would attend couple counselling in the future. Over half of both the autistic and non-autistic respondents answered yes to this question. This clearly shows that the majority of the couples who had attended couple counselling were still willing to try again despite some of the negative experiences they had endured. (For details of all responses to this question, please see Appendix 4.) However, the majority that answered yes to this question continued to state they would only attend couple counselling again if the counsellor was trained, knowledgeable and experienced in working with autistic neurodiverse couples.

The counsellor's experience and training in working with neuro-diversity were reported as the main reasons for the effectiveness or ineffectiveness of the counselling in the reports we received from both partners.

Following this question, the respondents were asked, 'How could couple counselling be improved when a partner has the characteristics of autism?'

This question is very relevant to the aim of this survey, as answers show the thoughts and recommendations of respondents who have had first-hand experience as a neurodiverse couple of a couple counselling setting. This question is seeking to discover what autistic neurodiverse couples really want from couple counselling.

The responses from both the non-autistic and autistic partners were of a very similar nature (explored in the previous chapters). We found that one keyword was used in over a quarter of all the responses from both groups: the word 'Understand/ing'.

(AFP) 'Counsellors MUST have intimate understanding of AS I think to be effective'.

(NAFP) 'In psychosexual understanding of AS'.

(NAFP) 'Therapist must understand AS in an adult with a new DX [diagnosis] and how it plays out in a relationship'.

The need to be understood as an individual and/or as a couple was expressed numerous times in the responses, as was the need for the counsellor to have an equal understanding of both partners in the relationship. This was highlighted as a necessary prerequisite for the success of any future counselling.

Lack of understanding by the counsellor was cited by both the autistic and non-autistic partners as one of the main reasons counselling failed them. Equally, being understood by the counsellor was stated as one of the principal reasons the couple's counselling proved beneficial and successful for respondents whose experience was positive.

Genuine empathetic responses by the counsellor cannot be offered without understanding. If a counsellor does not have any training or experience in what it means to be autistic and what it means to love and live with an autistic partner, then it is not possible for the counsellor to offer genuine empathy and understanding, to either partner.

Understanding is a very broad expression that encompasses a whole range of core conditions that a counsellor should be able to offer their clients in a genuine and caring way. The word understanding is synonymous with empathy, being considerate, kind, supportive, accepting and thoughtful. These are all the responses that a client would expect to receive from a counsellor and, in most cases, all the conditions that counsellors are trained to offer. However, if the counsellor is uninformed and untrained in working with autism and neurodiverse couples, these conditions will be difficult to meet, due to the lack of understanding the counsellor has of autism.

Understanding by the counsellor will only be achieved when adequate training and support are provided to couple counsellors; until that point, neurodiverse couples and individuals (Mitran, 2022) will continue to be denied the therapy they need. Mitran (2022) reported in her work as a licensed counsellor working with neurodiversity that 99% of her clients had reported one or more negative counselling experiences due to the therapist, counsellor or mental health provider being uninformed.

Similarly we have listened to numerous reports from the clients we have worked with over the years stating how they have been let down by the previous counselling they have received. Many clients were left with feelings of anger and humiliation by the counsellor's lack of understanding, training and knowledge.

> (AMP) 'It needs to be positive and work on strengths and respectful of the person and their thought process and not be patronizing'.

We have frequently witnessed in our work with autistic clients the relief expressed by both partners exclaiming how, for the first time, they felt understood. Mitran (2022) states that the reports she received from her clients clearly indicate the lack of skilled counsellors available who are able to understand how to support someone who thinks differently than the 'norm'. These findings are further supported by Camm-Crosbie et al. (2019) in their online survey for autistic adults. In addition, lack of training, skills and experience is not solely limited to counsellors; a study on neurodiverse couples also found the same lack of knowledge in other health professionals they encountered (Smith et al., 2020).

If the counsellor is uninformed and has not received any training in counselling neurodiverse couples, they are more likely to work with the couple as though they are non-autistic and will be blind to the differences that exist between them and each other. This will increase the likelihood of the counsellor having unrealistic expectations of the couple's ability to communicate together and their capacity to practise skills and coping strategies aimed at a non-autistic relationship. Some of these exercises would be totally inappropriate and hence cause further damage to what is often already a fragile and sensitive relationship. The need for both partners to be understood and given appropriate tools for coping is illustrated in the quotes below:

> (AFP) 'Less pressure on the AS partner to act non-autistic'.

> (AMP) 'The counsellor having a complete understanding of Asperger's

syndrome and not expect the person to be expressing emotion when they just don't know how'.

(NAFP) 'Give tools to each partner to help them communicate better. Help each person to understand how each other thinks and acts'.

Unless the counsellor is aware of and understands the needs of both partners, a feeling of equality and balance in the sessions will not be achieved. This could result in the counselling being unsuccessful. Training needs to encompass the perspectives of both partners in the relationship in equal measure.

(AFP) 'Provide tangible strategies to improve communication of feelings, understanding of my difficulties and challenges and how we as a couple can overcome them and both feel equal and equally have something positive to give/receive from the relationship and each other'.

(NAFP) 'By providing specific tools to couples. Perhaps some sort of regimen to follow in the case of a disagreement? Somehow it would have to be a process that would be respected by both couple members'.

(NAFP) 'Strategies to share daily life, balance intimacy, parent, setting boundaries for both partners to have time out or discuss issues would be more helpful'.

Respondents offered many practical suggestions for how future counselling could be improved. One of these was for separate sessions to be offered as well as couple sessions. Whilst one non-autistic partner suggested separate sessions for her autistic partner only, this recommendation came mainly from the autistic respondents in the survey. One of the reasons for this is the fear of confrontation. Some autistic individuals have a strong aversion, and many will do anything to avoid possible conflict, including remaining silent for fear of upsetting their partner. This fear will be the product of their life and relationship experience, as there will have been times that they gave the wrong response or said the wrong thing, often at an inappropriate time. This is likely to have resulted in their partner becoming upset or angry. The consequence of this is that they will say nothing at all. Unfortunately, without understanding and change, this may exacerbate the misunderstandings between the couple. Being offered a separate session, in a safe space, to talk without any pressure could be a lifeline to the autistic partner.

> (AMP) 'Encouraging the AS partner to analyse the situation can result in harmful statements that cannot be retracted. The AS partner must be encouraged to respond in emotional or empathetic terms. The important thing I need to learn is how to respond with empathy, or to mimic empathy convincingly. It seems that to effect empathy, I need to use different mental processes than a non-autistic person uses. When I try, I either fail altogether, or I fail to convince. Perhaps I need acting lessons'.

> (AFP) 'I would have welcomed some time with the counsellor individually to be able to express myself in a less pressurized environment. When my partner is there, I find I cannot be completely honest and am scared of his reactions'.

A need for longer sessions was also expressed. Maxine's sessions with clients were one and a half to two hours long. She discovered very early on that 50-minute sessions achieved very little and were too short for the longer processing time needed by autistic individuals to process emotional information. Tony has found that the sessions may include moments of silence as the autistic partner processes and adjusts to new information or interpretation without interruption or distraction.

> (NAFP) 'Longer appointments, more frequently, training for the AS person not to be hypersensitive about their poor skills. How to be teachable in the first place'.

If the couple counsellor is unaware of autism or has not been trained in communication that would be appropriate and beneficial with an autistic client, then the counsellor will base their communication style as though the client is non-autistic and will expect empathetic spontaneous responses. Therefore, questions such as 'and how do you think that makes your partner feel?' will be directed at the autistic client with the expectation that they will be able to offer a spontaneous response.

Just this question alone could result in causing both friction and anguish for both partners.

> (AMP) 'For a counsellor to speak our dialect of emotion...to be more challenging'.

Respondents in our survey also suggested that a need for alternative ways of communicating between the couple should be offered and taught by the counsellor. Encouraging note taking and summarizing sessions was suggested. Both these strategies are highly recommended in the *Good Practice Guide* published by the National Autistic Society working with Mind (2021). Tony sometimes encourages the couple to make an audio recording of the relationship counselling session on their mobile phone to facilitate accurate recall of the session.

> (AFP) 'A clear explanation of how the process would work, i.e. a person would be given the chance to speak without interruption and then the other would respond. A short summary of what we had covered at the end of the session would have been useful for me. I would like to have written down questions to think about during the week as I need time to process them'.

> (AMP) 'Explain and understand the different ways of communication. Allow and encourage note taking'.

The need for the counsellor to act as a translator between the couple is something that we have recommended to counsellors for many years and taught in our workshops. When exploring the support services available to neurodiverse couples, Smith et al. (2020) found the need for a counsellor to translate between each partner was raised as being crucial to the success of the counselling by one of their participants. The participant stated that counselling would be a 'waste of time' without this. The following response to our survey expresses this well:

> (AFP) 'I think there might have been more gain for me if the therapist had acted as a 'translator' to explain my difficulties to my husband, in a way that made sense to him and felt non-threatening. She could maybe have focused on some realistic goals to work with him to achieve'.

As well as a need for the counsellor to have a thorough understanding of what it means to be autistic, much emphasis in the reports was placed on the need for the counsellor to understand what it means to be the non-autistic partner in a neurodiverse relationship, and in particular the effects of Cassandra syndrome, also known as affective deprivation disorder. There will be further information on Cassandra syndrome in Chapter 10.

> (AMP) 'In my view Asperger's is an "issue" not a problem. The problem is denial about the issue and that really is the heart of the matter. The Cassandra syndrome issues really ring a bell with me'.

> (NAFP) 'The therapist would have to have knowledge of the reality of the (Cassandra) syndrome'.

> (NAFP) 'ALL Counsellors should be trained in AS and the effect on spouses'.

A need for counsellors to develop and be trained to have a better understanding of autistic women was expressed by two autistic female respondents. It is important for relationship counsellors to be regularly informed of the latest developments in our understanding of autism and neurodiverse relationships such as how an autistic partner may suppress and camouflage the characteristics of autism within a relationship.

> (AFP) 'Knowledge of the counsellor, especially differences of women on the spectrum'.

> (AFP) 'Therapist being aware for the challenges that ASD/non-autistic couples face, understanding the challenges of male but also FEMALE people on the spectrum'.

A need for counsellors to be trained to spot and identify the traits of autism was highlighted in the responses.

> (NAFP) 'Lots and lots of training to identify the signs. Helping couples to develop strategies to communicate better and deal with conflict in a way which addresses their unique perspectives'.

(AMP) 'Marriage counsellors should look for ASD. It took many years after this original counselling to be diagnosed. Had we realized at this point seven years ago, our marriage would probably not be now in name only. I think doing something is better than doing nothing, but it could have been SO much more if the counsellor had known how to look for Asperger's – just given me an AQ test'.

Smith et al. (2020) reported on the limitations of support available to neurodiverse couples and how at present the therapeutic approach employed by most relationship counsellors is of little benefit to neurodiverse couples. The results from our survey echo this and show the need for counsellors to be provided with adequate training and to be offered the knowledge and expertise they require to work with autistic neurodiverse couples. Only then will neurodiverse couples begin to receive the counselling services they deserve. Only then will they be given the same chance as non-autistic couples to save and potentially enhance their relationship, and avoid the devastation of a broken relationship.

Training, experience and understanding from a counsellor can make the difference between staying together or not for a neurodiverse couple. There are many positives to be gained from the coming together of differences in a relationship, but these positives are not always obvious to the couple; however, with genuine understanding, guidance and direction from a well-informed counsellor, unrealistic negatives can be turned into realistic positives. Good counselling can create new realistic expectations and healthy boundaries, teach self-care and personal responsibility and rebuild the love that brought the couple together in the first place. The response below is one of hope and deserves to be heard. Now is the time for professionals to listen, take notice and act.

(NAFP) 'Capitalizing on the gifts of these unique individuals and the joys they can bring each other...and acknowledging and supporting the additional loads for the non-autistic partner'.

REFERENCES

Camm-Crosbie, L., Bradley, L., Shaw, R., Baron-Cohen, S., & Cassidy, S. (2019). 'People like me don't get support': Autistic adults' experiences of treatment for mental health difficulties, self-injury and suicidality. *Autism, 23*(6), 1431–1441.

Mitran, C. (2022). Challenges of licensed counsellors and other licensed mental health providers working with neurodiverse adults: An instrumental case study. *The Family Journal.* https://doi.org/10.1177/10664807221123553

National Autistic Society & Mind. (2021). *Good practice guide*. https://s2.chorus-mk.thirdlight.com/file/24/asDKlN9as.klK7easFDsalAzTC/NAS-Good-Practice-Guide-A4.pdf

Smith, R., Netto, J., Gribble, N., & Falkmer, M. (2020). 'At the end of the day, it's love': An exploration of relationships in neurodiverse couples. *Journal of Autism and Developmental Disorders, 51*(9), 3311–3321. https://doi.org/10.1007/s10803-020-04790-z

Understanding Autism in a Relationship

CHAPTER 7

How to Recognize Autism in the Counselling Room

This chapter describes the signature characteristics of autism that may be apparent when first meeting a client or over several appointments when exploring their relationship history. The text is based on our extensive experience and the diagnostic criteria for autism spectrum disorder in the DSM-5-TR published by the American Psychiatric Association (2022).

PREVALENCE OF AUTISM

According to the Centers for Disease Control and Prevention (2024) in the United States, the prevalence of autism in 2023 was estimated as 1 in 36 eight-year-old children. However, this is a conservative estimate of the prevalence of autism, as many autistic individuals do not discover they are autistic until their adult years.

In early childhood, an autistic child will come to realize that they are different to their peers. They notice that their peers can easily and accurately 'read' social situations and people's thoughts, feelings and intentions, an ability that autistic children find elusive. There are also differences in interests, learning styles and sensory perception. An autistic child can have the personality characteristic of being an extrovert, wanting to connect and engage with their peers. Unfortunately, their social approaches to play and talk may be rejected, and they will often experience teasing, humiliation and bullying from their peers for being different.

A characteristic of autism is seeking patterns and systems which can be applied to social situations. An autistic child can be very sensitive and reactive to making a social 'error' and quietly observe their peers' play and social interactions from a discrete distance. Their intention is to imitate their peers. They become a 'child psychologist' exploring and analysing their peers' dynamics, personalities and social conventions. Once they have a 'script', they may be brave and launch themselves into social play, hoping to be accepted and liked. This process has been described as camouflaging autism or creating a 'mask' or alternative persona.

As adults, they may camouflage and suppress their autism at work or choose a career that minimizes the effects of autism, such as being self-employed or working alone at home in occupations such as data entry and analysis, graphic design or accounting. This is an effective form of autism compensation. Camouflaging and compensation may delay professional recognition of autism until the adult years.

SIGNS OF AUTISM

As the conversation with the client develops, the characteristics of autism may slowly emerge in their conversational abilities, social development, emotional communication, cognitive profile, ability to cope with change, interests and sensory sensitivity. A relationship counsellor may be the first person to recognize autism in a partner's developmental history and profile of abilities.

Conversation Abilities

The client's conversation ability, while often demonstrating sophisticated vocabulary and depth of knowledge, may also include subtle difficulties with the pragmatic aspects of language, unusual prosody, a tendency to make a literal interpretation, and difficulty with the comprehension and expression of non-verbal communication. The pragmatic aspects include the degree of reciprocity or 'balance' in the conversation: the person may talk too little or too much. When too little, there will need to be an encouragement to say more than a few words in reply to a question and to provide some degree of elaboration and personal examples that illustrate a specific topic. There can be a tendency for the non-autistic partner to talk for them, and it is important to allow the autistic partner to speak for themselves without interruption. When talking too much, the client's conversation may be perceived as a monologue. There can be difficulty in determining when the person has completed what they want to say; for example, failing to give eye contact to indicate it's your turn to speak. In addition, the autistic client may frequently interrupt their conversation partner to make a comment or correct an error, oblivious of the signals not to interrupt or that the person may be offended by the correction.

There may also be difficulties in knowing how to maintain and repair a conversation by seeking clarification and more information, and modifying language according to the social context. The client may also engage in too much or too little personal or confidential information disclosure.

Prosody may be unusual regarding the speed, volume, rate, rhythm and 'melody' of speech. There may be a lack of vocal tone and volume to indicate emotion and keywords, and an unusual placement of stress and precise intonation. There can be a tendency to take a literal interpretation, which may become apparent when their conversation partner uses idioms, sarcasm or 'figures of speech'.

One of the central characteristics of autism is difficulty focusing on and reading non-verbal communication, which can become conspicuous during a conversation. There may be difficulties in terms of eye contact frequency and duration, and ability to read another person's facial expressions in order to modify the conversation. The person may be listening but not looking at the face of their conversation partner at key points in the interaction when eye contact would be anticipated.

One of the adaptations to autism is to appear to be looking at the person's face, but instead focusing on their ears or forehead rather than the eyes, which communicate considerable emotional or conversational information. They may thus fail to determine what their conversation partner is feeling or communicating. Sometimes, even though there may be a focus specifically on someone's eyes, reading non-verbal communication from the area around the eyes can still be difficult. As one autistic adult said, 'People give messages with their eyes, and I don't understand them'.

The difficulty in reading non-verbal communication can occur for both conversation partners; the autistic client's facial expressions may be perceived as 'still' or 'wooden' and thus difficult to read. Their gestures may be limited or 'stylized', sometimes mimicking the gestures and posture of the conversation partner. There may be less use of nodding agreement, reciprocal smiles or sounds of compassion and gestures of interest. These are illustrations of the double empathy problem that will affect the relationship and conversation with a relationship counsellor.

Social Abilities and Experiences

During childhood, there is likely to have been a time when the client first recognized that their social and friendship skills were not as advanced as those of their peers. There may have been, and may continue to be, a preference for solitary rather than social activities. There may have been a desire to establish and maintain friendships throughout childhood and into the adult years without a complete or realistic idea of what friendship entails at each stage of development. Exploring social abilities and experiences may reveal a history of difficulty in making and keeping friends, one of the diagnostic criteria for autism.

Many autistic adults have experienced rejection, humiliation and bullying from peers, especially in their high school years. These incidents can be extremely distressing and traumatic. There is also an association between autism and all forms of abuse, which may lead to post-traumatic stress disorder (PTSD).

Expressions of Autism

A common perception of an autistic person is someone who considers social interactions as indecipherably complex, overwhelming and stressful and chooses to be alone but does not necessarily feel lonely. They may be perceived as an introvert, alone by choice. However, there are autistic adults who are highly motivated to engage socially and are extroverted, but who may not be able to read the subtle social signals and social conventions of what to say and do. A metaphor to describe this aspect of autism is that of a driver who does not see the traffic signals (non-verbal communication) or abide by the traffic code (social conventions). Their social behaviour may be perceived as intrusive or intense, such that the autistic person becomes bitterly disappointed that conversations, friendships and relationships are short-lived.

An adaptation to autism that creates the impression of social competence is for the person to acquire social abilities by suppressing their autistic characteristics and observing, analysing and imitating social behaviour, thus creating a social 'mask' and false persona. This adaptation is described as social 'camouflaging'.

While social success and acceptance may be achieved this way, the psychological cost is mental exhaustion in terms of being drained of mental energy by intellectually rather than intuitively processing social information. There is also the potential for the development of depression from energy depletion and the inability to express the authentic self.

When a marriage vow formalizes the relationship, the autistic person has achieved their objective and can, at last, express rather than suppress their autistic characteristics and be their authentic self. However, when first meeting a relationship counsellor, the autistic partner may revert to wearing their social mask, meaning the counsellor gains a false impression of their social and interpersonal abilities.

Another social adaptation or compensation for autism is for autistic girls and women to prefer the company of males since their social dynamics are relatively simpler. They may also feel safer and less likely to be judged negatively and rejected by males, who often enjoy interacting with a 'tomboy'.

A further adaptation is to develop an interest and talent in the arts, becoming an author, artist, musician or singer. Social eccentricities may be accepted and accommodated due to being valued by peers who recognize and admire a particular talent.

Alexithymia

Autism is associated with alexithymia, the inability to recognize and accurately communicate internal emotions and thoughts in spoken words. Alexithymia is not exclusive to autism or a characteristic of all autistic adults but has been identified in at least 50% of autistic adults and in only 5% of the general population (Kinnaird et al., 2019). Having alexithymia leads to difficulty recognizing internal emotional states, such that when asked 'What are you feeling now?', after some conscious thought, the reply may be, 'I don't know'. This is not being obtuse or evasive. There can be genuine difficulty in perceiving and converting internal states and emotions into speech. The full answer to the question would be, 'I don't know...how to mentally grasp the intangible emotions and thoughts swirling in my mind, identify and label them accurately and communicate them in speech so that you will understand'. The ability to perceive and accurately describe and disclose inner thoughts and feelings within a conversation is a central component of relationship counselling. The autistic client may have genuine difficulty converting their thoughts and feelings into speech.

Another characteristic of alexithymia is talking about experiences without reference to the emotional states of oneself and others. There is less spontaneous mention of emotions in conversation. This will affect autobiographical memory, such that an autistic client may describe an important event primarily by the sequence of actions rather than by the thoughts, feelings and intentions of others or themselves.

Empathy

Psychologists have conceptualized three forms of empathy. Cognitive empathy is the ability to determine what someone is feeling or thinking by 'reading' their facial expressions, gestures, vocal tone and the social context. An autistic person may need to use intellect rather than intuitive abilities to identify and process non-verbal communication they see and hear. Emotional empathy is the ability to 'feel' the emotions of others. A recurring theme from our experience of talking to autistic adults and reading autobiographies is an oversensitivity to the negative feelings of other people, such as disappointment, anxiety or agitation. Autistic individuals may mirror or amplify negative emotions in others (Fletcher-Watson & Bird, 2020). As one of the participants in that study said, 'We express empathy differently'. This has been described as empathy over-arousal (Smith, 2009) and occurs in autistic males and females (Schwenck et al., 2012). We have yet to determine how this ability is achieved, but quotations from autistic adults we have known may provide some indication:

> I am able to distinguish very subtle cues that others would not see, or it might be a feeling I pick up from them.

> There's a kind of instant subconscious reaction to the emotional states of other people that I have understood better in myself over the years.

While we have found that someone's negative mood can be 'contagious' for an autistic person, they may not be equally 'infected' by and absorb someone's positive mood. They can seem impervious to someone trying to 'cheer them up'. Happy and exuberant positive emotions in others may sometimes cause an autistic person to be confused and uncomfortable and not know how to respond or resonate with the joy of others, for example at a family celebration or reunion or when someone receives exciting news.

The third form of empathy is behavioural empathy, which is knowing how to respond to someone's feelings. Autism is associated with uncertainty in identifying what is expected to be said or done to alleviate or respond to someone's distressed feelings. An example would be giving their partner a hug and saying comforting words when they are upset. This can be a major cause of distress for both partners in the relationship. The autistic partner may be accused of lacking empathy. However, it is more a difficulty of 'reading' the subtle signals that indicate compassion or affection are anticipated, and intuitively knowing what to do.

Cognitive Abilities

Autism is associated with a cognitive profile that includes an ability to perceive and develop systems and patterns and also to identify errors and details that others may not recognize. There can be an ability to store and recall information from long-term memory and to find solutions to problems that are elusive to colleagues or employers. To think outside the box. This may lead to a successful career as a valued expert and problem solver in a particular career or profession.

Ability to Cope with Change

The diagnostic criteria for autism refer to insistence on sameness, inflexible adherence to routines and difficulty coping with change and transitions. For an autistic adult, variety is not the 'spice of life'. The autistic partner may describe needing considerable forewarning of a change to an anticipated routine, and their non-autistic partner has to accommodate the emotional reaction to change and uncertainty and difficulty coping with spontaneity.

Interests and Talents

Throughout childhood and into the adult years, an autistic partner often has a history of hobbies or interests that are unusual in intensity or focus. Each interest or passion has a 'use by date' that may range from hours to decades. The interests are associated with intense enjoyment and may also function as a thought blocker for anxiety or sadness. They also provide a sense of identity regarding being perceived as an expert and social connection with those who share the same interests.

During the conversation, the client may be somewhat subdued and quiet, appearing reluctant to engage. However, when the topic of conversation is the person's interest, they can suddenly become enlivened, engaged and eager to disclose their expertise – almost an alternative persona.

While alexithymia is a difficulty converting thoughts and feelings into speech, a successful adaptation to alexithymia is expressing thoughts and feelings through the arts. The autistic adult may have a recognized talent as an artist, musician, composer or author. The inner world of thoughts and feelings is vividly expressed through the arts, not conversation.

There may be a talent in the caring professions, especially psychology and psychiatry. The propensity from childhood to observe and analyse others to facilitate social engagement may evolve into achieving formal qualifications and a successful career as a teacher, therapist, psychologist, paediatrician or psychiatrist. Autism is often associated with the altruistic desire to educate and help alleviate suffering and injustice.

While autistic individuals have difficulty understanding and relating to people, they may have a talent for relating to animals. This can range from family pets to a career in veterinary science and zoology.

One autism myth is that some careers, such as the caring professions, would not be suitable for someone who is autistic. However, we have found that autistic individuals may have a successful career in all occupations or professions.

Sensory Sensitivity

One of the diagnostic criteria for autism is hyper- or hypo-reactivity to sensory experiences. An autistic person's sensory systems may be over- or under-responsive. Specific sounds, types of lighting, tactile experiences or aromas can be perceived so intensely that the experience is extremely aversive and to be avoided, or some sensory experiences are hardly noticed, such as enjoying extremely spicy or 'hot' food or not changing clothing to accommodate hot or cold weather.

There may also be difficulty sensing the internal world, or 'interoception', with what appears to be a mind and body disconnection. The autistic person may not experience hunger or thirst to the same degree as other people and may not be aware of the increasing heart rate and breathing that indicate rising anxiety or anger.

SCREENING FOR AUTISM AND CONSIDERING A FORMAL DIAGNOSTIC ASSESSMENT

At the end of the first consultation or after several consultations, the signs of autism may gradually become apparent to a relationship counsellor. The counsellor then has to decide whether or not to describe their perception of autism in one or both partners. In making that decision, it will be important to determine how that person will likely react to the counsellor's suggestion that they seek a formal diagnostic assessment and whether the diagnosis would benefit either or both partners and the relationship counselling.

If there are indications of a positive attitude to exploring autism as a factor in the relationship, the relationship counsellor could ask the client and their partner to complete screening questionnaires specifically designed to identify the characteristics of autism in an adult. These include:

- Autism Social Quotient (Baron-Cohen et al., 2001)

- GQ-ASD (Brown et al., 2020)

- CATI (English et al., 2021)

- AWE (Groen et al., 2023).

We have found that there can be considerable differences between each partner's perceptions of autistic characteristics as described in these screening instruments. If the partner who shows signs of autism disagrees with the suggestion that they are autistic, they may deliberately minimize their self-rating of autistic characteristics. If the non-autistic partner is convinced their partner is autistic and this provides the explanation they have been seeking for their relationship issues, they may magnify their partner's autistic characteristics. Our experience is that the greater the discrepancy between the partners' rating scores, the greater the disharmony in the relationship. Either way, if the scores on these instruments are above the designated cut-off, a referral for a formal diagnostic assessment may be warranted.

REFERENCES

American Psychiatric Association. (2022). *Diagnostic and statistical manual of mental disorders* (5th ed., text rev.). American Psychiatric Association.

Baron-Cohen, S., Wheelwright, S., Skinner, R., Martin, J., & Clubley, E. (2001). The autism-spectrum quotient: evidence from Asperger syndrome/high-functioning autism, males and females, scientists and mathematicians. *Journal of Autism and Developmental Disorders*, *31*(1), 5–17.

Brown, J., Attwood, T., Garnett, M., & Stokes, M. A. (2020). Am I autistic? Utility of the Girls Questionnaire for Autism Spectrum Condition as an autism assessment in adult women. *Autism in Adulthood*, *2*(3), 216–226.

Centers for Disease Control and Prevention. (2024). *Data and statistics on autism spectrum disorder*. www.cdc.gov/autism/data-research/index.html

English, M., Gignac, G. E., Visser, T. A. W., Whitehouse, A. J. O., Enns, J. T., & Maybery, M. T. (2021). The Comprehensive Autistic Trait Inventory (CATI): development and validation of a new measure of autistic traits in the general population. *Molecular Autism, 12*(1), 37.

Fletcher-Watson, S., & Bird, G. (2020). Autism and empathy: What are the real links? *Autism, 24,* 3-6.

Groen, Y., Ebert, W. M., Dittner, F. M., Stapert, A. F., Henning, D., Greaves-Lord, et al. (2023). Measuring the Autistic Women's Experience (AWE). *International Journal of Environmental Research and Public Health, 20*(24), 7148.

Kinnaird, E., Stewart, C., & Tchanturia, K. (2019). Investigating alexithymia in autism: A systematic review and meta-analysis. *European Psychiatry, 55,* 80-89.

Schwenck, C., Mergenthaler, J., Keller, K., Zech, J., Salehi, S., Taurines, R., Romanos, M., Schecklmann, M., Schneider, W., Warnke, A., & Freitag, C. M. (2012). Empathy in children with autism and conduct disorder: Group-specific profiles and developmental aspects. *Journal of Child Psychology and Psychiatry, 53*(6), 651-659.

Smith, A. (2009). The empathy imbalance hypothesis of autism. *The Psychological Record, 59,* 489-510.

CHAPTER 8

The Effects of Autism in a Relationship

Autism has many qualities that can be appealing to a potential partner. These include an intense passion for their interests, speaking their mind, being honest and having a strong sense of social justice. There can be technical or artistic abilities, good career prospects, and personality characteristics such as being kind and socially naive. They may have shared interests, sense of humour and moral values. Both partners may recognize characteristics they are familiar with in a parent or family member, which leads to a natural understanding and connection.

The autistic partner can be perceived as someone whose true social abilities will be unlocked and transformed by their non-autistic partner's social expertise. Indeed, their social expertise may be attractive to an autistic person because of their potential to be a social mentor.

Some couples share autistic characteristics, if not a formal diagnosis, in terms of preferring solitary rather than social pursuits, preference for routines and consistency, intense interests and sensory sensitivity. They may have both experienced peer rejection at school and have a deep mutual empathy for each other's past social and emotional experiences. They may feel more comfortable with someone who does not have great social expectations and does not seek frequent physical intimacy. Both partners have similar characteristics and expectations, so the relationship can be successful and enduring. However, from our experience, there may not be a perfect balance in relationship abilities and expectations, and they may seek relationship counselling to resolve specific issues.

The early stages of dating may not indicate to either partner the long-term relationship issues associated with autism. The autistic partner may have initially camouflaged and suppressed their autistic characteristics to be more attractive to a non-autistic partner. They may have acquired a dating 'script' from watching romantic movies and created a 'mask' or artificial persona. However, eventually, the mask is removed, and it becomes apparent that the autistic partner has difficulty with the intuitive understanding of how to maintain a long-term relationship.

Gradually, some of the emerging characteristics of autism can cause distress and conflict in the relationship, such as difficulty reading social cues, expressing feelings, the frequency of social experiences, emotion regulation and repair, expression of love and affection, intimacy, communication, conflict management and household responsibilities. These issues reflect many of the themes in conventional relationship counselling, but autism can affect the reasons why these issues have developed, and the relationship counselling will require modifications to accommodate autism.

READING SOCIAL CUES

Some of the issues in the relationship can be due to aspects of 'Theory of Mind', a psychological term that describes the ability to read facial expressions, body language, tone of voice and social context to determine what someone is thinking or feeling. Both partners experience this. We have known for some decades that autism is associated with Theory of Mind difficulties, which are part of the diagnostic criteria. However, we now recognize that the non-autistic partner can also have difficulty 'reading' the inner thoughts and feelings of their autistic partner. This is described as the double empathy problem (Milton, 2012). The autistic partner may not express subtle emotions in facial expressions, tone of voice and body language.

EXPRESSING FEELINGS

In a conversation, the autistic partner can struggle to find the words to express thoughts and feelings due to aspects of interoception and alexithymia (see Chapter 7). That is the sensory perception of the body signals that indicate emotional states such as heart rate and breathing (interoception) and being able to translate the emotions that you feel or remember into speech (alexithymia). This will affect the ability of the autistic person to disclose their inner world and communicate their feelings. As the relationship progresses, the non-autistic partner will anticipate increasing self-disclosure as a sign of the depth of the relationship and trust, not recognizing their partner's genuine difficulty in perceiving and communicating their inner world.

FREQUENCY OF SOCIAL EXPERIENCES

Autistic adults can achieve successful social engagement, but this may be by intellect rather than intuition, often with social guidance from the non-autistic partner or by consciously suppressing autistic character-istics and developing an alternative persona based on past observation and analysis of social situations, effectively camouflaging their autism. Thus, social occasions are mentally exhausting and energy-draining for an autistic partner. In contrast, the non-autistic partner may find that social experiences require little mental energy and may create energy.

The initial optimism that the autistic partner will gradually change and become more socially skilled and confident can dissolve into despair that social skills are static due to limited motivation and energy to be more sociable. The non-autistic partner may reluctantly agree to reduce the frequency and duration of social contact with family, friends and colleagues for the sake of the relationship but feel deprived of experi-ences they enjoy and find refreshing rather than exhausting.

The non-autistic partner may recognize that their autistic partner can engage socially at work but, on returning home, is exhausted and actively seeks solitude or engagement in a hobby or interest as a means of energy recovery. Although the couple lives together, the autistic partner may have a diminishing need for social, conversational and lei-sure time together. The autistic partner can be content with his or her own company for long periods of time. Although the couple are living together, conversations may be few and primarily involve the exchange of information rather than an enjoyment of each other's company, expe-riences and shared opinions. As one autistic partner said, 'My pleasure does not come from an emotional or interpersonal exchange'.

EMOTION REGULATION AND REPAIR

Autism is associated with experiencing strong emotions, especially anx-iety, anger and depression, and difficulty coping with stress at work and home (Attwood, 2006). There may be issues in the relationship regarding anxiety because the autistic partner can try to alleviate anxiety by being very controlling, and life for the whole family is based on rigid routines and predictable events. There may be concerns regarding anger management for both partners and the risk of physical and psychological abuse (Arad et al., 2022). Both partners may be vulnerable to being depressed (Arad et al., 2022; Gotham et al., 2015).

Anger management for both partners can be an issue in the relationship that leads to seeking relationship counselling. Autism is associated with difficulty perceiving the internal signals of increasing agitation due to aspects of interoception (see Chapter 7) and regulating the response according to the situation. The tendency is to become extremely angry quickly but to recover quickly. We recognize that a propensity to become angry for an autistic partner can be due to frustration from being thwarted from accessing strategies to reduce anxiety, such as playing a computer game or solitude. An emotional 'explosion' of anger or meltdown can be a means to discharge the emotional energy created by anxiety, or anger can be an unusual expression of depression. The depression is externalized rather than internalized, and the person goes into 'attack' mode rather than self-blame.

A non-autistic partner may express anger slowly and in stages. However, an autistic partner may not read the early signs of increasing agitation and not adjust their behaviour accordingly, which can escalate the situation. The non-autistic partner often expects emotional comfort to repair their distress, but gestures of love and affection may not be perceived by an autistic person as an automatic emotion repair mechanism, with a hug perceived as an uncomfortable squeeze which does not make them feel better. A typical comment of the non-autistic partner is that hugging their autistic partner is like 'hugging a piece of wood'. The person does not relax and enjoy such close physical proximity and touch.

Being alone is often the primary emotional repair mechanism for an autistic partner, and they may assume that is also the case for their non-autistic partner, with the thought that if they leave their partner alone, they will get over it quicker. They may also not know how to respond to their partner's distress or fear worsening the situation. In one relationship counselling session, an autistic partner sat next to his wife, who was in tears. He remained still and offered no words or gestures of affection for emotional repair. When asked if he was aware his wife was crying, he replied, 'Yes, but I didn't want to do the wrong thing'.

The autistic partner can be accused of being callous, emotionally cold and lacking empathy. However, this is due to a genuine difficulty reading interpersonal signals and intuitively knowing how to respond. The non-autistic partner gradually realizes that they need to be very clear and direct in expressing their feelings and suggesting to their partner what they need to do for emotional repair.

Surveys of the mental and physical health of couples where one partner is autistic indicate that the relationship has very different health effects for each partner (Arad et al., 2022; Aston, 2003). Most autistic male partners considered that their mental and physical health had significantly improved due to the relationship. They stated they felt less stressed and would prefer to be in the relationship than alone.

In contrast, most non-autistic partners stated that their mental health had significantly deteriorated due to the relationship. They felt emotionally exhausted and neglected, and many reported signs of clinical depression (Lewis, 2017). A sense of grief may be associated with losing the hoped-for relationship, as illustrated by the comment, 'It's not only what I've lost, it's what I've never had…' (Millar-Powell & Warburton, 2020). Most non-autistic survey respondents also stated that the stress associated with the relationship had contributed to a deterioration in physical health.

EXPRESSION OF LOVE AND AFFECTION

In a conventional relationship, regular expressions of love and affection are expected. A metaphor for the need and capacity for expressions of love and affection can be that a non-autistic partner has a 'bucket' capacity for love and affection that needs to be regularly filled and replenished. In contrast, an autistic partner has an affection 'cup' capacity that is quickly filled. The autistic partner may be perceived as not expressing sufficient affection to meet the needs of his or her partner, who feels affection-deprived and unloved, which can contribute to low self-esteem and depression.

When the autistic partner recognizes the value of expressions of love and affection in the relationship, there can be the issue of the frequency, type, intensity and duration of expressions of love and affection. As an autistic partner said: 'We feel and show affection but not enough and at the wrong intensity' and 'I know I am not meeting her needs, but I don't see them; will I ever be able to make my partner happy?'

While regular expressions of love and affection are powerful and effective means of emotional and energy replenishment for a non-autistic partner, an autistic partner may achieve replenishment through solitude and engagement with a hobby or interest rather than interpersonal experiences with their partner.

INTIMACY

There may be issues for both partners with verbal, emotional and physical intimacy. The effects of alexithymia (see Chapter 7) will inhibit the autistic partner's verbal and emotional intimacy, that is, converting thoughts and feelings into speech. However, an autistic partner may be able to express their thoughts and feelings indirectly using music, poetry, a scene from a movie, a passage in a book or typing rather than speaking their thoughts and feelings.

Sensory sensitivity may affect physical intimacy, leading to confusion, distress and frustration with sexual experiences for an autistic partner (Gray et al., 2021). Autism is associated with a low or high threshold for sensory experiences, especially tactile experiences. A low threshold can lead to experiencing discomfort or pain when lightly touched during moments of intimacy. A high threshold can lead to requiring greater physical stimulation, as in the comment from the Gray et al. study, 'I am not particularly sensitive, so I need more friction to achieve orgasm' (2021, p. 5). There may also be the issue of the use of drugs and alcohol, as in another comment from the same research study, 'Only when I am drunk do I feel comfortable being touched or touching others' (p. 6).

There can be issues with the frequency and quality of physical intimacy, which influences sexual satisfaction (Bolling, 2016). Sex can become an intellectual interest for an autistic partner in acquiring information on sexual diversity and activities, often from pornography, and sex may function as a means of self-calming and emotion regulation. This was described by one of the participants in the Gray et al. (2021, p. 5) study: 'I went through this highly sexualized phase because I just loved the way orgasms made me feel and connected me to myself and centred me. It was like the best self-regulation strategy I had found' (p. 5). The non-autistic partner may not reciprocate the desire for and frequency of sexual activities and experiences.

However, from our extensive experience, the non-autistic partner is more likely to be concerned about the lack of sexual desire rather than an excess. The autistic partner may become asexual once he or she has children. In a relationship counselling session, the partner of an autistic man was visibly distressed when announcing that she and her husband had not had sex for over a year. Her autistic husband appeared confused and asked, 'Why would you want sex when we have enough children?'

COMMUNICATION

As the non-autistic partner describes their daily experiences, their autistic partner may not engage in the anticipated degree of eye contact and words, sounds and gestures of compassion and interest. The autistic partner absorbs the story but does not appear attentive and is eager to provide practical advice rather than non-judgemental listening and empathy. Non-autistic partners may feel they lack emotional support but experience considerable practical advice.

A communication issue in a relationship where one partner is autistic is a tendency for the autistic partner to be perceived as overly critical and correcting and rarely providing compliments. The autistic partner intends to improve their partner's proficiency and anticipate gratitude for their advice, being unaware of the effect on their partner's self-esteem. There may also be a reluctance to provide compliments due to not intuitively knowing that in a relationship, the non-autistic partner needs frequent approval and admiration. There is also the factor that sometimes the autistic partner is reluctant to give a compliment when their partner is already aware of their achievement.

We have also found that the autistic partner may feel emotionally uncomfortable when given a compliment due to being unsure how to respond and whether what they did or said warrants a compliment.

CONFLICT MANAGEMENT

In any relationship, there will inevitably be areas of disagreement and conflict, but there is usually a range of strategies used by both partners to resolve conflict. Effectiveness in resolving conflict is a significant factor in relationship satisfaction for both autistic and non-autistic partners (Bolling, 2016). One of the consequences of difficulties with Theory of Mind and the double empathy problem is misinterpreting intentions, such as determining whether a comment or action was deliberately malicious, humorous or benign. This can lead to either partner being quick to take offence.

Unfortunately, an autistic partner may not be skilled in the art of clarification, negotiation, accepting alternative perspectives, compromise and apology. There can also be difficulty accepting even partial responsibility. Non-autistic partners may complain, 'It is never his/her fault', or, 'I always get the blame'. There can also be an inability to show remorse, to forgive and forget, and often ruminating on past miscommunication and criticism. The autistic partner may have had limited experiences of childhood and adolescent friendships where conflict management strategies are discovered, practised and enhanced.

HOUSEHOLD RESPONSIBILITIES

In modern Western society, we have replaced the words 'husband' or 'wife' with the word partner. This reflects changing attitudes towards long-term relationships. There is an expectation of sharing the workload at home, for domestic chores and caring for the children, and being each other's best friend regarding the disclosure of thoughts and feelings, reciprocal conversation, sharing experiences and emotional support. Taking on the role of a best friend is not easy for an autistic partner due to having lifelong difficulties making and maintaining friendships.

The majority of autistic adults have problems with executive function, that is, organizational and time management abilities, distractibility and prioritization, procrastination and completing tasks (Rosello et al., 2022). The non-autistic partner may realize they need to take disproportionate responsibility for the family finances, ensuring jobs are completed and resolving the organizational and interpersonal problems that have developed in their partner's work situation. The non-autistic partner takes on the role of executive secretary, frequently prompting their partner on what to do (Wilson et al., 2014). This aspect of the relationship adds to the stress and responsibility of the non-autistic partner and the autistic partner feeling undervalued and misunderstood.

DEVELOPMENTAL HISTORY

Autistic adults are often 'late developers' in terms of social and emotional maturity and friendship and relationship knowledge. Friends may have been few and far between, and there may have been a lack of interpersonal experiences, confidence in their relationship skills, and subsequent low self-esteem.

The majority of autistic adults will have suffered peer rejection, bullying and humiliation throughout childhood and adolescence. They may also have experienced trauma and abuse from peers. An additional factor can also be a history of not being understood and supported by a range of professionals, from teachers to psychiatrists. These aversive experiences and a lack of effective support and therapy will affect their sense of trust and create the belief that relationship counselling is futile. The non-autistic partner may have had to take some time encouraging their partner to attend the initial relationship counselling session.

Unfortunately, autistic adults may not be able to intuitively identify the relationship 'predators' in life and may not be wise in their choice of partner. They may have been the victim of abuse in previous relationships. They may initially feel compassionate and caring for their partner and cannot extricate themselves from a history of being attracted to malevolent characters who recognize their low self-esteem, vulnerability and gullibility. As one autistic woman explained, 'I set my expectations very low and, as a result, gravitated towards abusive people. I cannot stress the importance of recognizing how important self-esteem is to an autistic adult'.

AUTISTIC BURNOUT

An autistic life is not an easy life. There is the potential for great stress and chronic exhaustion from trying to cope with social and sensory experiences, being misunderstood and criticized, high levels of anxiety and, for many reasons, not feeling in touch with or able to be the authentic self. In addition, self-imposed expectations may be greater than coping mechanisms and abilities. Subsequent stress can build up over time, which can lead to autistic burnout, characterized by increased social withdrawal, a form of 'hibernation' and reduced executive functioning; the frontal lobes are 'closed', awaiting recovery.

When considering whether a partner has autistic burnout, it is important to review the similarities and differences between autistic burnout and depression. In comparison to the signs of depression, in autistic burnout, there is increased sensory sensitivity and the need to isolate in order to recover. The current clinical and experiential wisdom is that autistic burnout is a cause of depression and that depression is likely to be reduced if measures are taken to resolve the causes of burnout. Autistic burnout can last months or years and may start in the adolescent years.

The relationship is likely to have included several episodes of autistic burnout, which may be triggered by life changes such as starting a new job or promotion or having children. One of the central characteristics of autistic burnout and depression is a depletion of energy, which could affect the ability to respond to relationship counselling.

THE DISCOVERY OF AUTISM

Either partner may have become aware of the characteristics of autism from the diagnosis of a child in the family or information on autism available in the media. This can lead to a revelation that autism may be an explanation for some of their relationship issues.

Some recent research has been investigating online forums and lay literature exploring the experience of discovering a partner is autistic (Lewis, 2017). Six themes emerged:

1. Facing unique challenges within the relationship

2. Insisting partners seek a diagnosis

3. Initial shock and relief

4. Losing hope for 'normalcy'

5. Making accommodations within the relationship

6. Wishing for professional support.

Relationship counselling can address all six themes.

REFERENCES

Arad, P., Shechtman, Z., & Attwood, T., (2022). Physical and mental well-being of women in neurodiverse relationships: A comparative study. *Journal of Psychology & Psychotherapy*, *12*, 420. https://doi.org/10.21203/rs.3.rs-955119/v1

Aston, M. (2003). *Asperger's in love: Couple relationships and family affairs.* Jessica Kingsley Publishers.

Attwood, T. (2006). *The complete guide to Asperger's syndrome.* Jessica Kingsley Publishers.

Bolling, K. M. (2016). *Asperger's Syndrome/Autism Spectrum Disorder and marital satisfaction: A quantitative study.* PhD dissertation, Antioch University, New England. https://aura.antioch.edu/etds/257

Gotham, K., Unruh, K., & Lord, C. (2015). Depression and its measurement in verbal adolescents and adults with autism spectrum disorder. *Autism*, *19*(4), 491–504.

Gray, S., Kirby, A. V., & Graham Holmes, L. (2021). Autistic narratives of sensory features, sexuality, and relationships. *Autism in Adulthood, 3*(3), 238–246.

Lewis, L. F. (2017). 'We will never be normal': The experience of discovering a partner has autism spectrum disorder. *Journal of Marital and Family Therapy, 43*(4), 631–643.

Millar-Powell, N., & Warburton, W. A. (2020). Caregiver burden and relationship satisfaction in ASD-NT relationships. *Journal of Relationships Research, 11*, e15.

Milton, D. E. M. (2012). On the ontological status of autism: The 'double empathy problem'. *Disability & Society, 27*(6), 883–887. https://doi.org/10.1080/09687599.2012.710008

Rosello, R., Martinez-Raga, J., Mira, A., Carlos Pastor, J., Solmi, M., & Cortese, S. (2022). Cognitive, social, and behavioral manifestations of the co-occurrence of autism spectrum disorder and attention-deficit/hyperactivity disorder: A systematic review. *Autism, 26*, 743–760.

Wilson, B., Beamish, W., Hay, S., & Attwood, T. (2014). Prompt dependency beyond childhood: Adults with Asperger's syndrome and intimate relationships. *Journal of Relationships Research, 5*, e11.

CHAPTER 9

The Adaptations for Autism in a Relationship Counselling Session

Many aspects of autism need to be considered and accommodated during a relationship counselling session. These include terminology, sensory sensitivity, interoception, alexithymia, the ability to read non-verbal communication, language profile and executive functioning abilities.

TERMINOLOGY

It is important that the relationship counsellor is aware of recent developments regarding person-first or autism-first language. Professionals have previously been encouraged to use person-first language, that is, 'the person with autism'. However, the autistic community now prefers autism-first language, that is, the autistic person. At the start of the first relationship counselling session, if one or both partners has an autism diagnosis or consider themselves as autistic, it would be wise to know the client's preferred term so as not to cause offence.

SENSORY SENSITIVITY

Autism is associated with auditory, visual, tactile and olfactory sensitivity. The Sensory Perception Questionnaire (SPQ) was designed to confirm and explore the sensory sensitivity of autistic adults (Tavassoli et al., 2014). The questionnaire includes descriptions of extraordinary sensory sensitivity, such as:

I can hear electricity humming in the walls.

I notice the flickering of a desktop computer even when it is working properly.

I would be able to hear the sound of a vacuum cleaner from any room in a two-storey building.

I cannot go out in bright sunlight without sunglasses.

I close the curtains to avoid bright lights.

It is important to consider the sensory aspects of the relationship counselling room regarding autistic sensory sensitivity. There may need to be a variety of illumination and light intensities, as well as being aware of the distraction of a clock ticking, a chair scraping on the floor and voices from another room. Consideration may be given to switching off electrical equipment that is not needed during the counselling session and choosing different seating choices. It may be wise to avoid potentially aversive olfactory experiences such as perfumes, aftershave and scented deodorants. There may also be a sensitivity to the room's temperature, with a preference for cool temperatures. Sensory modifications to the counselling room can reduce the distractions and discomfort of sensory experiences and stress.

INTEROCEPTION AND ALEXITHYMIA

An autistic client may have difficulty with interoception, which is cognitive awareness of bodily sensations such as increasing heart rate, breathing and muscle tension that indicate rising anxiety, agitation or despair. There is almost a mind-and-body disconnection and difficulty making sense of the body's internal signals unless they are clear and strong. This will affect the autistic person's ability to perceive and effectively regulate and communicate low levels of emotion to their partner and the relationship counsellor. Thus, internal emotional states seem to fly under the mental radar and tend to build up and may eventually be released in an emotional meltdown, which is distressing to both partners and the relationship counsellor. The mind/body connection can be enhanced by the relationship counsellor recommending activities such as yoga, meditation and mindfulness in daily life.

The term alexithymia describes a characteristic associated with but not exclusive to autism, namely an impaired ability to identify and describe thoughts and feelings in speech. The prevalence of alexithymia in autistic adults is around 50%, while the prevalence in the general population is 5% (Kinnaird et al., 2019). Alexithymia is associated with difficulty focusing on and accurately appraising the subtleties and textures of internal emotional states. As one autistic adult said, 'I'm not good at wording my feelings'.

When asked, 'How are you feeling about this?' an autistic client with alexithymia may answer, 'I don't know'. They are not being evasive or obtuse; they may have genuine difficulty describing inner thoughts and feelings using spoken language. Their reply could continue to, 'I don't know... how to grasp in my mind the feelings I am experiencing, "hold" a specific feeling and then determine the word or phrase that precisely describes that feeling'.

For example, an autistic woman described all negative feelings that she experienced as 'ick'. On further discussion of what 'ick' meant, she could not say anything more than it was a 'bad' feeling, and she did what she could to avoid it. As we explored the context for one of her descriptions of feeling 'ick', it was clear that she had experienced embarrassment, but the precise word was elusive. Difficulty identifying what you are feeling will inhibit the ability to regulate the feeling.

Another consequence of alexithymia is a tendency for those who have it to focus on external rather than internal experiences and to mention thoughts and emotions less spontaneously in conversation with their partner and the relationship counsellor. We have frequently noted that alexithymia can interfere with engagement and progress in relationship counselling, where there is an expectation of the ability to accurately perceive, disclose and resolve feelings. When feelings and thoughts are not easily disclosed, there can be an interpretation that thoughts and feelings are being deliberately suppressed or avoided rather than them being difficult to articulate in speech.

There are screening questionnaires such as the Toronto Alexithymia Scale (Bagby et al., 1994) that can assess and confirm alexithymia. The Toronto Scale explores three dimensions of alexithymia: identifying feelings, describing feelings and externally orientated thinking. Another questionnaire is the Perth Alexithymia Questionnaire (Preece et al., 2018). This questionnaire includes negative and positive emotions. If alexithymia is confirmed, this will be valuable information for the relationship counsellor to explain how alexithymia can affect the relationship and relationship counselling.

Strategies exist to reduce the effects of alexithymia during counselling sessions. For example, the 'wheel of emotions' is available on the internet. An external prompt, seeing the word in print, may facilitate finding the words to describe feelings.

Within the relationship, an autistic partner may be able to and encouraged to express feelings by typing rather than talking, such as sending their partner an email or using the arts to express their feelings. For example, they may write a poem, choose a music track that describes their feelings in the music or lyrics, or choose a passage or scene from a favourite book or film that portrays the emotion.

The association between alexithymia and autism is well-documented. Tony created the term alexipersona to explain the characteristics of a limited vocabulary for describing personality. In conversation with an autistic partner, the relationship counsellor may notice they seem to have few words to describe personality characteristics or personality types in others and themselves. The relationship counsellor may consider assessing personality traits to help the autistic partner's self-understanding and to explore the concept of personality in themselves and their partner.

READING NON-VERBAL COMMUNICATION

A non-autistic partner will likely be astute at perceiving and understanding non-verbal communication. Their mind prioritizes social cues above other information in their environment, and they intuitively understand what non-verbal communication, social cues and context mean and how to respond.

The relationship counsellor needs to recognize that an autistic client has genuine difficulty reading non-verbal communication or cognitive empathy and knowing intuitively how to respond with words and gestures of compassion and affection—that is, behavioural empathy. It is not an absence of empathy, with the implication that the autistic client does not care about the feelings of others. The autistic partner probably does care very profoundly but may not be able to identify and 'read' the more subtle signals of emotional states and respond as anticipated by their partner. An interpretation of this characteristic is to assume that the autistic partner is being callous, malicious or manipulative. However, the autistic partner is often unaware rather than dismissive of their partner's feelings.

As the non-autistic partner describes their distressing experiences within the relationship, observation by the relationship counsellor of the autistic partner's facial expressions and body language may not indicate they sympathize with or have compassion for their partner's feelings. This may be an expression of the double empathy problem in that it may be difficult for the non-autistic partner or relationship counsellor to read the autistic partner's non-verbal communication. Their facial expressions may be difficult to read and sometimes almost 'frozen'. The stillness may not be due to indifference but can be due to taking time to process social information and determine what to do. An autistic adult explained that there can be a delay in deciding which face and gestures to make in the situation. They can also appear unusually serious during moments of levity and laugh a fraction of a second after everyone else in the room due to a delay in cognitively processing social information.

LANGUAGE ABILITIES

The signature language profile associated with autism needs to be accommodated within a relationship counselling session; for example, the counsellor being aware of the autistic client's propensity to make a literal interpretation and thus avoiding idioms, figures of speech and sarcasm. It is essential to be clear and avoid ambiguity. There can also be issues with narrative ability when describing events, such as keeping to the point, giving too much or too little information and being pedantic. Another concern can frequently be interrupting the counsellor to correct a trivial error, or having something to say and being unable to wait or else the comment will be quickly forgotten. Autism is also associated with difficulties with conversation reciprocity, potentially dominating the conversation or being reluctant to contribute to the conversation.

A language quality associated with autism is the ability to use metaphors to visualize a concept. The relationship counsellor can actively use metaphors. We have found that metaphors based on the autistic person's interests or passions can be particularly effective.

EXECUTIVE FUNCTIONING ABILITIES

Research suggests that between 40 and 70% of autistic adults also have impaired executive functioning (Rong et al., 2021), which can include difficulties prioritizing and sustaining attention, limited organizational skills, distractibility, impulsivity and difficulty conceptualizing and considering potential and alternative outcomes, and completing activities within the expected time frame. Their partner may have reluctantly taken on the role of executive secretary in their daily life.

Impaired executive functioning will also affect the relationship counselling session, as breaks will be needed to accommodate the autistic client's attention span and ensure that the room is clear of distracting clutter. The relationship counsellor may consider explaining the structure and schedule for the current and subsequent sessions to clarify what is expected and needed, including completing activities described during the session at home and their executive secretary partner to help them remember to complete relationship assignments.

An aspect of autistic executive functioning difficulties is cognitive rigidity, that is, having a 'one-track mind' and difficulty considering alternative perspectives and responses. These alternatives may need to be stated explicitly rather than assumed to be understood intuitively. Once an ability is acquired, an autistic adult may still require someone to prompt them about what to do and when. In a relationship, the autistic person's partner may be distressed because they frequently have to remind their autistic partner to initiate the relationship strategies agreed upon with the relationship counsellor. This could be perceived as lacking commitment to the counselling, but may actually be due to aspects of impaired executive functioning.

A relationship counselling session is probably a new experience for an autistic adult. Explaining the therapeutic relationship and ground rules for the counselling sessions may be valuable for all participants. This can include not being distracted by phone calls and social media, contact outside of counselling sessions, confidentiality and trying not to interrupt when someone is talking.

Autistic clients are likely to complain that the sessions involve too much talking. The cognitive profile associated with autism can include poor auditory working memory, and it may help the autistic partner to process and remember key points if they are able to make notes or have a workbook. The learning profile can also include a preference for achieving new abilities by reading rather than conversation. The relationship counsellor may suggest literature for the autistic partner to read to clarify, augment and consolidate the key points from a counselling session.

Another characteristic of autism is slow processing time. The relationship counselling session will require the autistic partner to process new information and responses within the relationship. The relationship counsellor may need to be silent and not interrupt the autistic client as they process new information during the relationship counselling session.

REFERENCES

Bagby, R. M., Parker, J. D. A., & Taylor, G. J. (1994). The twenty-item Toronto alexithymia scale. *Journal of Psychosomatic Research, 38*, 23–32.

Kinnaird, E., Stewart, C., & Tchanturia, K. (2019). Investigating alexithymia in autism: A systematic review and meta-analysis. *European Psychiatry, 55*, 80–89.

Preece, D., Becerra, R., Robinson, K., Dandy, J., & Allan, A. (2018). The psychometric assessment of alexithymia: Development and validation of the Perth Alexithymia Questionnaire. *Personality and Individual Differences, 132*, 32–44.

Rong, Y., Chang-Yiang, Y., Yang, Y., Jin, Y., & Wang, Y. (2021). Prevalence of attention-deficit/hyperactivity disorder in individuals with autism spectrum disorder: A meta-analysis. *Research in Autism Spectrum Disorders, 83*, 101759.

Tavassoli, T., Hoekstra, R. A., & Baron-Cohen, S. (2014). The Sensory Perception Quotient (SPQ): Development and validation of a new sensory questionnaire for adults with and without autism. *Molecular Autism, 5*, 29. https://doi.org/10.1186/2040-2392-5-29

CHAPTER 10

Cassandra

THE HISTORY BEHIND CASSANDRA

The first time the name Cassandra was brought to our attention in relation to the experience of the non-autistic partner was when we both spoke at the 'Families of Adults Afflicted with Asperger Syndrome' (FAAAS) Conference held in Cape Cod, USA, in 2000. The late Karen Rodman organized the conference for FAAAS. Cassandra syndrome had previously been named 'mirror syndrome' by the FAAAS organization. This name was chosen as it was observed that the non-autistic partner would, over time, in a long-term relationship, mirror the traits of autism. The mirrored traits were mixed but mainly appeared as socially withdrawing, communicating less and suppressing emotions.

Rodman (2003) published a collection of contributors' personal accounts, information and submissions worldwide. Her book included the first published accounts from non-autistic women in neurodiverse relationships who identified 'Cassandra phenomenon' as a condition affecting the non-autistic partner in a neurodiverse relationship.

Rodman ends the chapter 'Cassandra phenomenon' with the words: We are 'the invisible walking wounded. We are Cassandra' (Rodman, 2003, p. 23).

We are often asked 'Why did the name Cassandra come to be applied this way?' In mythology, Cassandra was a prophetess, and the god Apollo was besotted with her. As a token of his love, he gave her the gift of prophecy, and she could foresee the future. However, the feelings were not mutual, and when Cassandra did not return his love, he became resentful and cursed her never to be believed.

According to the story of Cassandra, she went on to make many prophecies, but no one ever took her seriously, and she died disregarded and unbelieved. The non-autistic women in the FAAAS group strongly identified with feelings of not being believed. Many described how they had spent years trying to describe to their friends, family and professionals how they felt and what they experienced within the relationship, and no one took them seriously or listened. Hence the title of Rodman's book, *Asperger's Syndrome and Adults... Is Anyone Listening?*

Over the past two decades, the Cassandra phenomenon has been renamed Cassandra syndrome, Cassandra affective disorder, Cassandra affective deprivation disorder (Aston, 2007a) and affective deprivation disorder (Aston, 2007b). More recently, the label 'ongoing traumatic relationship syndrome' has been used to describe the effects of Cassandra syndrome. For ease of use, we will use the term Cassandra syndrome as this was the original term used first to describe the non-autistic partner when in a state of being unacknowledged and disbelieved.

Today, Cassandra syndrome has become a common term and appears within the chapters of many books written over the past two decades on the subject of autism and relationships (Arad, 2020; Bentley, 2007; Holgate, 2024; Jones, 2023; Moreno et al., 2012; Rodman, 2003; Simone, 2009; Wilson, 2022). In addition, support groups, blogs and information regarding Cassandra syndrome are now easily available on the internet.

The characteristics of Cassandra syndrome are more likely to develop when a couple are unaware that they are neurodiverse or, although aware, do not accept or understand what being neurodiverse means for each of them and their relationship.

Our survey found many mental and physical health symptoms being reported by the non-autistic respondents, such as depression, low self-esteem, hopelessness and questioning one's sanity. Marital conflict has been found to lead to an increase in depression directly. It is shown to be a significant risk factor for physical and psychological health, particularly in midlife and older adults (Choi & Marks, 2008). Some of the respondents also reported that these symptoms increased after the counselling that the couple had received due to the non-autistic partner not feeling believed or validated by the counsellor. This supports the need for recognition not only of one partner as autistic but also of the effect of this on the non-autistic partner.

Cassandra syndrome is not due to any intentional behaviour from either partner and does not develop overnight. It builds slowly and can take many months or years to become apparent. Cassandra syndrome is situational, and once the couple becomes aware, accepts and understands they are neurodiverse, appropriate measures by both partners can be taken to alleviate the effects altogether. Understanding and acceptance can greatly improve relationship satisfaction for both partners. Feeling cared for and understood by a partner was shown to be associated with a lower negative affect in a longitudinal study conducted by Slatcher and Selcuk (2015). This study found that after ten years, the lower negative affect experienced by the partner was linked to healthier diurnal cortisol profiles. In contrast, adults who did not feel understood or cared for by their partner reported poorer well-being and reacted more emotionally to daily stressors (Stanton et al., 2019).

The leading cause of problems in Cassandra syndrome is that the very people who should be giving the couple support – family, friends, their partner and professionals – do not believe and take the non-autistic partner seriously. Although the original concept of Cassandra syndrome was based on the experiences of non-autistic female partners, the concept can be applied to all gender expressions of a non-autistic partner.

When a couple first turns to counselling services for support, it is often after many years of struggles and failed attempts by the couple to work it out for themselves. The couple may have reached a point of marital burnout or exhaustion trying to mend and resolve the misunderstandings and conflicts between them. Couple counselling is often the last resort, not the first, as it requires time and commitment and comes at a financial cost.

Going to see a couple counsellor is more likely to be initiated by the non-autistic partner (Holmes, 2023), and it may have taken a long period of prompting for the autistic partner to agree to go. To seek out and arrange to see a counsellor takes a great deal of courage from both partners, particularly the autistic partner. Venturing into the unknown, meeting someone new, changing routines and having to spend time communicating about some very personal topics can feel like the autistic partner's worst nightmare. Taking that first step is very bold and shows the level of commitment held by many autistic partners to the relationship, as well as a desperate desire to resolve the issues and end the conflict between them.

Unfortunately, if it is unknown to the couple that one partner is autistic, then this reluctance to seek support and help for the relationship will be interpreted by the non-autistic partner as uncaring, avoidant and unwilling to try to make the relationship work. This, in turn, will cause frustration, anger and feelings of loneliness for the non-autistic partner, which will exacerbate symptoms of depression and hopelessness, which were reported in the responses in our survey.

When the couple first arrive in the counselling room, the non-autistic partner may appear very emotional, frustrated and angry, and it would be easy to interpret their behaviour as aggressive and uncooperative. The part the counsellor plays in the sessions is often critical to the future of the relationship. If both signs of autism and Cassandra syndrome are passed over and not addressed or recognized, it is highly likely that the counselling will only serve to exacerbate the problems the couple are experiencing.

More research is required to explore further what Cassandra syndrome is and precisely what causes it. We know the autistic partner does not intentionally cause their partner to feel they are not believed. We also know that this feeling is not limited to those in an autistic relationship. It can also be due to living with a partner who is alexithymic. We do know from the research available and numerous books on the topic that not being understood or believed can seriously affect the mental and physical well-being of the non-autistic partner. And indeed this applies to both partners in the relationship: both need to feel validated, believed and understood, not just by their partner but by the professionals they are seeking support from.

A RELATIONAL DISORDER?

Cassandra syndrome has been classed as a relational disorder (Mendes, 2015; Simon & Thompson, 2009). The DSM-IV (APA, 1994, p. 737) refers to this under the heading 'Partner Relational Problem', and it is defined as 'persistent and painful patterns of feelings, behaviour, and perceptions, involving two or more partners in an important personal relationship'. Unfortunately, 'relational disorder' was deleted from the DSM-5 and subsequent revision DSM-5-TR.

What is very relevant in the case of a relational disorder is that it is not about the individual partners; it is caused by the relationship they share between them. Two perfectly healthy people who can both live an independent and healthy life without difficulties, can, when together, find themselves sharing an unhealthy relationship.

A relational disorder can occur in any type of relationship. In the case of an autistic neurodiverse relationship, this means that both partners will be processing social information differently, have different ways of communicating and have a different set of priorities and needs. If, as was the case in many of the respondents to our survey, the couple are not aware of or do not understand the difference between them, then they will have unrealistic expectations about each other. Neither will understand the other and due to the double empathy difficulty, neither will read or interpret each other accurately.

If the counsellor is not trained to identify the signs of autism or Cassandra syndrome, then they will be working with the couple as though they are both non-autistic and will have unrealistic expectations of what is achievable by the couple. The counsellor will also be unable to offer them understanding and validation. Therefore, the counsellor will not be able to offer beneficial strategies and make positive improvements to the relationship. Counselling will not educate the couple to understand each other and alleviate the feelings of blame and guilt that many couples experience.

Being in a neurodiverse relationship without the knowledge and understanding of what this means will affect both partners, who will be struggling to understand each other. Research has found that it is more likely to be the non-autistic partner who is in distress in the couple relationship (Smith et al., 2020) in comparison to the autistic partner who, as we saw in Strunz et al. (2017), reported higher scores on marital satisfaction than their non-autistic partner. There has been a significant link found between depression and marital dissatisfaction (Beach, 2014), and if the difficulties go unresolved, this leads to marital burnout. Marital burnout can occur when coping strategies employed to overcome and resolve the causal stress are ineffective (Ferri et al., 2015). Studies have found that in a relationship, marital burnout is more likely to affect women than men (Çapri & Gökçakan, 2013; Pamuk & Durmuş, 2015; Pines et al., 2011).

One of the reasons women are more likely to suffer from depression and marital burnout is thought to be due to their initially higher expectations of the relationship (Çapri, 2008). Non-autistic partners may have expectations at the beginning of the relationship that are unrealistic. This is more likely to be the case if it is unknown that one partner is autistic, and studies have found that if autism is not discovered or diagnosed till much later in the relationship then marital dissatisfaction is reported at higher rates (Strunz et al., 2017). This is due to the couple being unaware that their neurological differences are the factor which is causing the challenges and difficulties they are experiencing and preventing them from finding a mutual resolution.

Unrealistic expectations held by the non-autistic partner could have also developed if the autistic partner was masking in the initial stages of the relationship. Masking is when autistic individuals attempt to hide or camouflage their authentic selves for fear that the non-autistic population will not accept them. This masking can be particularly prevalent when attempting to form a relationship with a potential non-autistic partner. Autistic individuals may go to extreme lengths to mask any autistic traits when dating; this could include researching and observing and analysing non-autistic behaviour, consciously making eye contact, suppressing reactions indicative of being autistic, or adjusting communication style. Descriptions of remaining silent, not talking about oneself or one's special interests and trying to understand and talk about other people's interests were all reported in a study by Hull et al. (2017). Autistic individuals will often go to great lengths to ensure that dates go smoothly. One autistic gentleman described how he would prepare for a date by visiting the selected restaurant the evening before. He would inspect the seating plan to choose and book his preferred table and reduce the possibility of experiencing sensory overload from noise and movement.

The effort made can be very exhausting for the autistic individual and cannot be maintained long term without detrimental effects on their mental, physical and emotional health (Hull et al., 2017). The need for masking will often cease when the relationship becomes secure due to the couple moving in together or marriage. For the non-autistic partner, this is often when their expectations for relationship intimacy will be at their highest. This sudden change in their partner's behaviour and responses will be confusing and bewildering, leaving the non-autistic partner desperately trying to regain the attention and emotional responses they were receiving and enjoyed previously.

In an attempt to get their need for reciprocal interaction met, the non-autistic partner has been found to use prompts within their daily communication with their partner (Wilson et al., 2014). Some success has been found in using prompts; however, having to use prompts to initiate interactions and responses, would, over time, feel like more responsibility being placed on the non-autistic partner's shoulders. This added responsibility resulted in reports of feeling the relationship resembled a parent/child relationship, along with feelings of frustration, anger, loneliness and depression (Wilson et al., 2014).

WHAT ARE THE SIGNS AND SYMPTOMS OF CASSANDRA SYNDROME THAT A COUNSELLOR NEEDS TO BE AWARE OF IN THE NON-AUTISTIC PARTNER?

Below is a list of the symptoms that have been found by researchers to affect the non-autistic partner or have been reported by the non-autistic partner when in a neurodiverse relationship:

- A loss of sense of self (Wilson et al., 2017)

- Anger (Deguchi & Asakura, 2018; Lewis, 2017)

- Anxiety (Deguchi & Asakura, 2018)

- Confusion (Bostock-Ling et al., 2012; Lewis, 2017)

- Depression (Arad et al., 2022)

- Emotional depletion (Wilson et al., 2017)

- Exhaustion (Wilson et al., 2017)

- Feeling blamed (Deguchi & Asakura, 2018)

- Frustration (Bostock-Ling et al., 2012)

- Health issues (Arad et al., 2022; Wilson et al., 2017)

- Hopelessness (Bostock-Ling et al., 2012; Lewis, 2017)

- Loneliness (Bostock-Ling et al., 2012; Deguchi & Asakura, 2018; Wilson et al., 2017)

- Loss of hope (Lewis, 2017)

- Low subjective well-being/self-esteem/self-concept (Arad et al., 2022; Bostock-Ling et al., 2012)

- Low physical well-being or physical depletion (Arad et al., 2022; Bostock-Ling et al., 2012; Wilson et al., 2017)

- Low mental well-being (Arad et al., 2022)

- Mood disorders (Bostock-Ling et al., 2012)

- Repressed emotions (Deguchi & Asakura, 2018)

- Self-doubt (Deguchi & Asakura, 2018)

- Social isolation (Bostock-Ling et al., 2012; Deguchi & Asakura, 2018; Wilson et al., 2017)

- Stress (Lewis, 2017).

To recognize Cassandra syndrome in a client, the counsellor must be conscious of how the non-autistic partner presents in the counselling room. This can be divided into three components of awareness: what the counsellor is hearing, what the counsellor is observing and finally what the counsellor is feeling. We will explain each component below.

What the Counsellor Is Hearing from the Non-Autistic Partner

The most common question we hear in the counselling room from the non-autistic partner is 'I am going mad? Am I crazy? Am I losing my sanity?' This was also raised by the respondents in our survey and reported by participants in a study conducted by Wilson et al. (2017).

If someone casts doubt on another individual's reality, then the individual concerned will eventually doubt that reality. If that someone is a professional who is looked up to as the 'specialist' in these matters, then the doubt cast will be even more effective. This will be very similar to 'gaslighting', although in this case due to lack of knowledge rather than intentional harm.

Many respondents in our survey raised the feeling of not being believed by the counsellor which resulted in a very negative impact on the therapeutic relationship and in many cases on the couple's relationship too. If the effect of Cassandra syndrome is to be reduced, then the counsellor's recognition and validation of both partners is paramount, and offering this will result in a positive and stronger therapeutic alliance.

Complaints regarding exhaustion, burnout and excessive responsibility should be taken seriously by the counsellor and explored further. If possible, arranging an individual session for each partner may allow uninhibited dialogue that will allow the counsellor greater insight into the issues being experienced.

Reports regarding lack of change in the relationship, communication breakdown and confusion may also be expressed by the non-autistic partner before and during counselling. A counsellor is also likely to hear how confused the non-autistic partner feels by their partner's behaviour. The counsellor may be told their partner just 'doesn't get it'. This may be said in reference to the relationship difficulties being experienced, understanding how the non-autistic partner feels, and why what they are doing upsets their non-autistic partner so much. This could all be quite different from what the counsellor will be hearing from the autistic partner, who may be totally unaware of why their partner is so upset or angry.

What Behaviour Will the Counsellor Be Observing in the Non-Autistic Partner?

Unfortunately, for some neurodiverse couples by the time they make it into the counselling room, the non-autistic partner is often at the end of their tether and the presenting behaviour could include outbursts of anger and frustration alternating with crying and displays of intense emotion. This behaviour could be the direct opposite of the behaviour shown by the autistic partner, who, in contrast, may appear quite calm and genuinely confused by why their partner is so upset or angry. The autistic partner is sometimes hopeful that the counsellor will be able to sort out the issues and put things right.

It can be useful for the counsellor to acknowledge the discrepancy between the couple's presentations and reflect this back to the couple so that each may have time to consider and explore this theme in more depth with the counsellor.

What the Counsellor May Be Feeling

Intuition. A sense that something is missing or does not quite make sense. A counsellor may be aware of the confusion in the room and may, due to transference, find themselves also confused. Communication between the couple may not flow and appear as though the couple are talking in different languages without being aware of it. The counsellor may have the feeling that this is a couple that is not communicating or relating to each other from the same place. It can feel as though the couple's stories and recall of the same incident are so far removed from each other that it is as though they were in different places. Hence, feelings of confusion will be amplified.

This takes us back to working from a client's frame of reference, and here the counsellor will be presented with two very different frames of reference to manage that may often be in opposition to each other. All these are signs that the counsellor is working with a neurodiverse couple who are not aware of how differently their minds are working. This will need to be addressed and an individual counselling session for each partner should be offered if the couple feel that would work for them. This will allow each partner the time and freedom to express their own individual perspectives. This way the counsellor will be able to hear both perceptions and opinions and assess whether this is a neurodiverse couple and if one partner is autistic and whether the other partner is presenting with Cassandra syndrome. The counsellor will need to acknowledge both partners' stories and offer acceptance and understanding.

Regardless of the terminology used to describe Cassandra syndrome, it is very real for the individual who is experiencing it. A counsellor should discuss with their client what they would like to call it. Giving this condition a name gives it context, reality and meaning. Both partners will be able to explore and research further into what it means and why it occurs, just as they will be exploring and researching further into what being autistic means. The journey of discovery and recovery may work as a project of bonding for the couple and encourage both to understand each other's perspective and reality. Unlike being autistic, Cassandra syndrome is transitional and situational, and a full recovery with the appropriate support and incentive from both partners can be achieved. The result of this will be a healthier and closer relationship based on mutual respect for both partners.

REFERENCES

American Psychiatric Association. (1994). *Diagnostic and statistical manual of mental disorders: DSM-IV* (4th ed.). APA.

Arad, P. (2020). *When your man is on the spectrum: To know, understand & transform your relationship*. eBookPro Publishing.

Arad, P., Shechtman, T., & Attwood, T. (2022). Physical and mental well-being of women in neurodiverse relationships: A comparative study. *Journal of Psychology and Psychotherapy, 12*(1), 1000420.

Aston, M. (2007a). *Cassandra affective deprivation disorder.* www.maxineaston.co.uk/cassandra

Aston, M. (2007b). *Affective deprivation disorder.* www.maxineaston.co.uk/cassandra/AfDD.shtml

Beach, S. R. H. (2014). The couple and family discord model of depression: Updates and future directions. In C. R. Agnew & S. C. South (Eds.), *Interpersonal relationships and health: Social and clinical psychological mechanisms* (pp. 133–155). Oxford University Press. https://doi.org/10.1093/acprof:oso/9780199936632.003.0007

Bentley, K. (2007). *Alone together: Making an Asperger marriage work*. Jessica Kingsley Publishers.

Bostock-Ling, J., Cumming, S., & Bundy, A. (2012). Life satisfaction of neurotypical women in intimate relationships with an Asperger's syndrome partner: A systematic review of the literature. *Journal of Relationships Research, 3*, 95–105.

Çapri, B. (2008). *Investigation of attachment and emotion regulation characteristics on the prediction of married individuals' couple burnout*. Mersin Üniversitesi Sosyal Bilimler.

Çapri, B., & Gökçakan, Z. (2013). The variables predicting couple burnout. *Elementary Education Online, 12*(2), 561–574.

Choi, H., & Marks, N. F. (2008). Marital conflict, depressive symptoms and functional impairment. *Journal of Marriage and Family, 70*(2), 377–390.

Deguchi, N., & Asakura, T. (2018). Qualitative study of wives of husbands with autism spectrum disorder: Subjective experience of wives from marriage to marital crisis. *Psychology, 9*, 14–33. https://doi.org/10.4236/psych.2018.91002

Ferri, P., Guerra, E., Marcheselli, L., Cunico, L., & Di Lorenzo, R. (2015). Empathy and burnout: An analytic cross-sectional study among nurses and nursing students. *Acta bio-medica: Atenei Parmensis, 86*(Suppl 2), 104–115.

Holgate, C. J. (2024). *The mind boggling discovery of a difference: A love story*. Austin Macauley Publishers.

Holmes, S. (2023). Exploring a later-in-life diagnosis and its impact on marital satisfaction in the lost generation of autistic adults: An exploratory phenomenological qualitative study. *Global Journal of Intellectual & Developmental Disabilities, 12*. https://doi.org/10.19080/GJIDD.2023.12.555829

Hull, L., Petrides, K. V., Allison, C., Smith, P., Baron-Cohen, S., & Mandy, W. (2017). 'Putting on my best normal': Social camouflaging in adults with autism spectrum conditions. *Journal of Autism and Developmental Disorders, 47*, 2519–2534. https://doi.org/10.1007/s10803-017-3166-5

Jones, D. (2023). *The Aspie book*. Austin Macauley Publishers.

Lewis, L. F. (2017). 'We will never be normal': The experience of discovering a partner has autism spectrum disorder. *Journal of Marital and Family Therapy, 43*(4), 631–643. https://doi.org/10.1111/jmft.12231

Mendes, E. A. (2015). *Marriage and lasting relationships with Asperger syndrome*. Jessica Kingsley Publishers.

Moreno, S., Wheeler, M., & Parkinson, K. (2012). *The partner's guide to Asperger syndrome*. Jessica Kingsley Publishers.

Pamuk, M., & Durmuş, E. (2015). Investigation of burnout in marriage. *International Journal of Human Science, 12*, 162.

Pines, A. M., Neal, M. B., Hammer, L. B., & Icekson, T. (2011). Job burnout and couple burnout in dual-earner couples in the sandwiched generation. *Social Psychology Quarterly, 74*(4), 361–386.

Rodman, K. (2003). *Asperger's syndrome and adults... Is anyone listening? Essays and poems by partners, parents and family members of adults with Asperger's syndrome*. Jessica Kingsley Publishers.

Simone, R. (2009). *22 things a woman must know if she loves a man with Asperger syndrome*. Jessica Kingsley Publishers.

Simon, H. F., and Thompson, J. R. (2009) *Affective deprivation disorder: Does it constitute a relational disorder?* http://affective deprivation.blogspot.co.il

Slatcher, R., & Selcuk, E. (2015). Perceived partner responsiveness predicts diurnal cortisol profiles 10 years later. *Psychological Science, 26*. doi:10.1177/0956797615575022.

Smith, R., Netto, J., Gribble, N., & Falkmer, M. (2020). 'At the end of the day, it's love': An exploration of relationships in neurodiverse couples. *Journal of Autism and Developmental Disorders, 51*(9), 3311–3321. https://doi.org/10.1007/s10803-020-04790-z

Stanton, E., Selçuk, A. K., Farrell, R. B., & Slatcher, A. D. (2019). Perceived partner responsiveness, daily negative affect reactivity, and all-cause mortality: A 20-year longitudinal study. *Psychosomatic Medicine, 81*(1), 7–15.

Strunz, S., Schermuck, C., Ballerstein, S., Ahlers, C., Dziobek, I., & Roepke, S. (2017). Romantic relationships and relationship satisfaction among adults with Asperger syndrome and high-functioning autism. *Journal of Clinical Psychology, 73*(1), 113–125. https://doi.org/10.1002/jclp.22319

Wilson, B. (2022). *Have they gone nuts? The survival guide to social interaction in neurodiverse (autistic-neurotypical) relationships*. Privately published.

Wilson, B., Beamish, W., Hay, S., & Attwood, T. (2014). Prompt dependency beyond child-hood: Adults with Asperger's syndrome and intimate relationships. *Journal of Relationships Research*, 5, e11. https://doi.org/10.1017/jrr.2014.11

Wilson, B., Beamish, W., Hay, S., & Attwood, T. (2017). The communication 'roundabout': Intimate relationships of adults with Asperger syndrome. *Cogent Psychology*, 4(1), 1283828. https://doi.org/10.1080/23311908.2017.1283828

CHAPTER 11

What the Non-Autistic Partner Needs from Relationship Counselling

Responses to the survey clearly indicated that the non-autistic partner needs to be validated by the relationship counsellor and to be given explanations of how autism affects the relationship and appropriate adaptations for both partners.

VALIDATION

As the relationship develops, the non-autistic partner will become increasingly disappointed that the relationship is not as anticipated. While this disappointment can occur in many relationships, some aspects of a neurodiverse relationship may not be experienced by other couples. When the non-autistic partner discloses their concerns, it may become apparent that the autistic partner is unaware of those issues in the relationship and denies that they exist. As far as they are concerned, the relationship is working well, and their partner's concerns are insignificant. The non-autistic partner may then disclose their concerns to their family and friends, trying not to appear disloyal to their partner. They may not experience validation and compassion as the issues usually occur in private at home and may not have been noticed by family and friends. They may be sceptical or critical of the non-autistic partner, with unhelpful suggestions such as 'Just accept it' or 'You have a new Mercedes; what more do you want in a relationship?' The responses of their partner, family and friends can lead the non-autistic partner to question their insight, interpretation and sanity. Non-autistic partners often seek validation of their thoughts, feelings and reactions from a relationship counsellor. They anticipate non-judgemental listening, recognition of their experiences, compassion and validation of their concerns.

ADAPTATIONS IN THE RELATIONSHIP

Both partners will make adjustments and adaptations within the relationship to meet their partner's needs, but the non-autistic partner may feel that there is an imbalance as they have had to make more changes and adaptations than their partner. An example is reducing socializing with family and friends as the autistic partner finds such situations exhausting.

A characteristic of autism is the need for consistency in daily routines, the creation of rules and the insistence that others follow them, such as the 'correct' way to load the dishwasher, and the intolerance of any deviation from the rule. The autistic partner may genuinely believe that having set meals for each day of the weak is also their partner's choice rather than a reluctant accommodation to maintain peace and tranquillity at home.

The non-autistic partner will value and need expressions of love and affection as their preferred and most effective emotional restorative. However, the autistic partner may prefer engaging in a solitary interest as their preferred emotional restorative and may not perceive subtle signals that indicate they need to attend to their partner's distress, and if they do respond, it may be by withdrawing so that they can feel better by being alone because that is what works for them. The non-autistic partner often adapts by not anticipating the emotional repair that occurs in conventional relationships, which may result in low self-esteem and depression.

Gradually, the non-autistic partner will 'mirror' their autistic partner's behaviour, lifestyle and thinking to survive in the relationship. The 'trading of traits' may be perceived as a one-way trade. They are aware of why and how they have adapted to living with an autistic partner, as seen in the comments, 'I have developed into the person necessary for him' and 'The essential me had disappeared.' There is a grief reaction for no longer being who they were, feeling they are lonely in the relationship, and the stress is affecting physical and mental health. These adaptations will need to be validated by a relationship counsellor.

EXPLANATIONS

The non-autistic partner needs explanations for why their autistic partner thinks and behaves in unconventional ways. They may ask the relationship counsellor questions such as why does my partner:

Not Socialize with Me at Home as They Do with Their Colleagues at Work?

A non-autistic partner can reduce stress and feel refreshed at the end of the working day by disclosing their experiences, thoughts and feelings at work with their partner. A problem shared is a problem halved, and sharing experiences and a partner's compassion and affection are effective energy restoratives.

Successful socializing for an autistic adult is often achieved by intellect rather than intuition. Socializing at work can be exhausting, and when returning home, more socializing, even with a partner, can lead to further energy depletion. An autistic partner often needs solitude to restore energy levels. This is not the rejection of their partner but a need for solitude to intellectually process the working day and achieve energy restoration through a solitary activity such as engaging in computer games or a hobby such as painting figurines or using the internet to discover interesting information on butterflies. The non-autistic partner may delay conversation time in the evening until their autistic partner's energy levels are restored.

Need Me to Organize and Plan Their Day? My Partner Couldn't Organize Getting Drunk in a Brewery

The majority of autistic individuals also have some executive functioning difficulties associated with ADHD (see Chapter 16). These include difficulties with organizational and planning skills, time management, deciding priorities and completing tasks. They may need an executive secretary, in the past a parent and now a partner. This may be an onerous role for the non-autistic partner who has difficulty accepting that someone of such intellectual ability needs guidance and prompting for so many activities of daily living.

The relationship counsellor may explore the autistic partner's executive functioning skills and if difficulties are confirmed that affect the relationship, suggest the couple seek a diagnostic assessment for ADHD by a clinical psychologist or psychiatrist. If confirmed, various treatment strategies exist, including medication and mobile phone apps that can reduce reliance on a partner acting as an executive secretary.

Not Know How to Resonate with My and Others' Happiness?

A central characteristic of autism is difficulty with social and emotional reciprocity. When other people are feeling exuberant, an autistic person may not be able to absorb and resonate with their happiness. They may be unsure how to respond and feel more emotionally comfortable when other people do not express strong emotions, either negative or positive. They may be notorious in the family for dampening others' excited energy and being pessimistic. The relationship counsellor will often need to explain this characteristic as an expression of autism, and an autistic partner and the family may benefit from the non-autistic partner guiding their autistic partner in what to do or say when they or others are jubilant.

Have to Always Correct Me and Rarely, if Ever, Compliment Me?

One of the cognitive qualities of autism is the ability to identify errors. This is valuable in a work setting in design, problem solving and quality control. However, constantly correcting a partner can be a cause of relationship conflict. The intention may not be to make their partner feel stupid and themselves superior. The intention may be benevolent in wanting to improve their partner's abilities, and they are often unaware of how offensive this may be from their partner's perspective. Their focus is on improving their partner's abilities, not making them feel incompetent.

While criticism may be frequent, compliments may be rare. As one autistic partner said, 'Why should I compliment you for something you know you are good at?' A relationship counsellor may explain the importance of exchanging compliments in a relationship and ask the couple to review how often they give and receive compliments to enhance the relationship.

Need Me to Remind Them What to Say or Do to Help Me Feel Better?

There are many ways to repair emotions in a relationship. Often, a non-autistic partner's first choice is interpersonal, in terms of words and gestures of affection and compassion, which are perceived as the most effective and efficient. An autistic partner has probably always been confused in interpersonal situations, which can include emotional repair by actions such as a hug. As one autistic adult said, 'How can a hug solve the problem?' and 'Why would squeezing me make me feel better?' The emotional repair mechanisms often chosen by an autistic partner may be solitude, to await the natural reduction of feelings, as in the comment 'I wait until the storm has passed', or distraction (thought blocking), or an emotional antidote such as the pleasurable experience of engaging in a passionate interest. The autistic perspective may be that people are the cause of, not the solution to, an autistic person's emotional distress. This often seems like an alien concept for non-autistic partners.

Thus, interpersonal emotional repair mechanisms may not be their first thought. An autistic partner may deliberately walk away when their partner is distressed, not due to callous indifference but to facilitate what they see as an emotional restorative, solitude, thinking their partner will appreciate being left alone when distressed, or saying 'Just try not to think about it'.

The relationship counsellor can explain both partners' perspectives and, with mutual understanding, encourage the autistic partner to ask what they could do when their partner needs emotional repair. When this occurs, the non-autistic partner can express gratitude, which will give the autistic partner more confidence in using the same response again.

Explode with Anger? There Are Times When I Feel Scared and Vulnerable

Cognitive moderation of intense emotions can be difficult for autistic adults. Due to problems with interoception (the perception of internal body signals), they may not be cognitively aware of their signs of increasing agitation, such as increased breathing, heart rate and muscle tension. A partner may become aware of increasing signs of agitation such as increased speech volume, agitated arm gestures and contorted facial expressions. However, if the autistic partner is not cognitively aware of the signs they're displaying, they may be denied, and their non-autistic partner may be accused of misreading them.

Eventually, the build-up of emotional energy is released physically, which can be extremely frightening for all family members and pets. The discharge of emotional energy can lead the autistic partner to at last feel emotionally relieved. Subsequently, anger explosions can occur again due to the psychological concept of negative reinforcement, which is when an action to end an unpleasant state of mind works, and so is repeated. 'I feel better now' is a powerful reinforcement of the behaviour. While the autistic partner is now calm, the non-autistic partner can take some time to recover from the experience, and apologies may not be forthcoming or sufficient to resolve their distress and apprehension that this behaviour will occur again.

A relationship counsellor can validate the non-autistic partner's perspective and reactions and explore strategies to prevent and manage anger explosions with both partners. However, there may be a point when anger management issues in a relationship need to be addressed by a clinical psychologist.

Not Connect with Me as When We Were Dating?

An autistic adult may have developed the ability to consciously suppress and camouflage their autistic characteristics and create a social 'mask'. When dating, they may follow the script they have learnt from watching romantic movies or TV shows. They know their autism may not be perceived as a good quality by a potential partner, and they may delay the disclosure of their authentic self to strengthen the early stages of the relationship during dating.

Another characteristic of autism is intense passions or interests. We tend to think of these passions in terms of an intense focus on a hobby such as astronomy or collecting rare Beatles recordings. The focus can also be a person, perhaps a famous historical figure, but it can also be someone they know, such as someone for whom they have romantic feelings. There can be a degree of adulation and interest that is intense and intoxicating for the person they are dating, especially if the person they are dating has experienced limited interest and attention from previous romantic partners.

The suppression of autism may have a 'use by date', and the authentic self may become apparent when the relationship is formalized. The early adulation and focus of attention created memories of an enjoyable time in the relationship for the non-autistic partner. Their lament can be that their autistic partner was once able to demonstrate remarkable relationship skills, but this was an act, an artificial self. They may complain that if their partner could connect so well when dating, why do they have difficulty connecting now? A relationship counsellor can explore the quality of the relationship in the early stages, what might be retrieved from those times, and improve communication and connection for both partners.

Not Express Inner Thoughts and Feelings to Me?

We have previously described alexithymia (Chapter 7) as a characteristic associated with autism. This is difficulty converting thoughts and feelings into speech. This is not an evasive action but, as described earlier, a genuine problem that affects relationships and relationship counselling. There is another characteristic of autism that is not being able to intuitively know what a partner needs to or would like to know. As the relationship progresses, the non-autistic partner may gradually reveal past experiences for greater mutual understanding and trust. But the autistic partner may have difficulty with disclosing past events, sometimes due to trauma, but also due to alexithymia. As one non-autistic partner said, 'His mind is a book with secret chapters whose content will never be revealed'.

We have found that for some autistic partners, over- rather than under-disclosure can also be an issue, such as describing how good sex was with an ex-partner. There may be limited recognition that some things are better not disclosed. The relationship counsellor may encourage the autistic partner to consider what information is likely confidential or sensitive to their partner and to think about those thoughts but not say them, as this would upset their partner.

Never Seem to Be Listening to What I Say?

When someone is listening to their conversation partner, there is the expectation of frequent eye contact with the person who is talking. An autistic partner may be listening but not looking. Eye contact is needed to read facial expressions and body language, but an autistic partner may primarily focus on what is being said and have difficulty reading non-verbal communication, which can be confusing rather than clarifying. Concentration on what is being said is improved by looking away. The autistic partner is not following social conventions but may be absorbing what is said. The relationship counsellor can explain that their autistic partner is not expressing indifference or lack of respect but is using a constructive means of focusing, processing and remembering what their partner is saying, especially if they have limited verbal working memory and can quickly forget what was said.

Not Know How to Appreciate My Perspective and Resolve Disagreements with Compromise?

A central characteristic of autism is difficulty perceiving alternative perspectives. This is a combination of difficulty reading non-verbal communication (Theory of Mind abilities) to determine that someone has different thoughts, perceptions and beliefs, and cognitive rigidity in terms of a 'one-track mind', not 'seeing thoughts on other tracks' and being able to 'switch tracks'.

There can also be issues with compromise, which is based on an appreciation of different perspectives, finding common ground and a reasonable and realistic outcome. The art of compromise is often learnt through friendships in childhood and adolescence, and the autistic partner will probably have had limited previous experience of constructive conflict resolution and compromise. The relationship counsellor may explain constructive ways of managing disagreements and the value of reaching a compromise.

Think Our Relationship Is Fine When It Clearly Isn't?

This may be another example of difficulty perceiving an alternative perspective. The relationship may meet many of the needs of the autistic partner, significantly improving their quality of life, and there can be the assumption that the relationship adequately meets their partner's needs. However, this might not be the case with the non-autistic partner, who is often the one to seek relationship counselling. This can be resisted by the autistic partner who does not recognize any concerns that need a relationship counsellor and does not perceive the need to change as everything is fine. This conceptualization of the relationship was confirmed in our survey.

Not Understand Why I and the Children Need So Many Friends?

Non-autistic children and adults thrive on social experiences. They are motivated to seek and maintain friendships. Autistic children and adults can socialize, but engaging with friends is achieved by intellect rather than intuition, which is energy-depleting. Recovery is often through solitude. Home is their castle, and there can be resentment when friends and extended family members visit the home as they have 'invaded the sanctuary'.

The relationship counsellor can explain both perspectives and seek a compromise, which may include the non-autistic partner having a social life that does not include their autistic partner. This can be a satisfactory outcome for both partners. The children may have friends at their home when the autistic parent is not at home or is able to access a private sanctuary within the home.

Ruminate for Decades Over Past Injustice?

Injustice can be being bullied, teased, rejected or humiliated, or some-one not following an accepted social rule and code of conduct and get-ting away with it. Events may be replayed in thoughts and dreams, and closure may be elusive due to not understanding why someone would behave or act that way and there being no justice. Ruminating over being bullied may last decades, and the events may not be put into per-spective. The degree of distress is refreshed with each flashback. The relationship counsellor may recognize the signs of trauma and suggest accessing appropriate therapy.

Consider or Accept Being Autistic?

Some people in the general population, and some professionals, still consider autism a mental disorder. The Diagnostic and Statistical Man-ual of Mental Disorders defines the diagnostic criteria. There may be an understandable rejection by an autistic partner of being considered as having a mental disorder when, in society's terms, they are successful in their career and relationship and do not need psychiatric services or government support. The autistic partner has a point.

Another inhibitory factor in accepting being autistic is having an autistic family member and not identifying positively with that person. 'How dare you think I am like...'.

The relationship counsellor can focus on the qualities of autism in a relationship, explore and clarify the partner's negative perception of the diagnostic term, and encourage a paradigm shift in terms of the conceptualization of autism and how acceptance can contribute to an enhanced relationship for both partners.

CONCLUSION

To answer these questions, the relationship counsellor will need exten-sive training in autism and how it affects relationships. The counsellor will also need to be able to answer the non-autistic partner when they ask: 'What can change, what is unlikely to change, and how can we encourage change?'

CHAPTER 12

Understanding the Challenges That Face the Autistic Partner in a Relationship

It was only three decades ago when it was presumed by some profession-als that autistic adults were unlikely to have the skills or the desire to form romantic relationships, let alone maintain long-term relationships and have a family. This unjust and very inaccurate myth was fortunately soon discredited due to the overwhelming evidence from real-life cases.

Studies have found that autistic individuals can have both the desire for romantic relationships and the ability to form and maintain long-term relationships (Strunz et al., 2017). In their study, Strunz et al. found that 166 (73%) of their 229 autistic participants reported being in or having been in a romantic relationship. Of the group that was not in a romantic relationship, more than 50% expressed that they were afraid of not being able to meet a partner's demands. Their findings further showed that autistic adults who formed a relationship with another autistic individual reported higher relationship satisfaction.

TWO AUTISTIC PARTNERS

Our experience and research studies indicate that the satisfaction rate in autistic couples is higher than in neurodiverse couples, so they may be less likely to require the services of relationship counselling. This could possibly be the reason why we did not receive many responses from couples who were both autistic in our survey.

Our survey included responses from 41 autistic adults; of these only four (three females and one male) stated that their partner was also autistic. Two reported a positive outcome to the counselling and two a negative outcome. Both couples in the positive outcome were fortunate enough to have seen a counsellor that was trained in autism; this was not the case in the two negative outcomes.

In a study which involved 12 autistic individuals, Crompton, Hallett et al. (2020) found that autistic people felt more at ease and comfortable in the company of others who were also autistic and were able to achieve a stronger sense of belonging. The participants also expressed that they felt able to offer other autistic people more patience, understanding and empathy than they felt they could offer non-autistic people. Of these 12 individuals, ten were female. In our work with neurodiverse couples, we have both found that autistic women, rather than autistic men, were more likely to choose a partner who was also autistic. This is certainly a subject which would benefit from further exploration and research in the future.

Relationships between two autistic individuals have been reported as experiencing a higher relationship satisfaction than individuals in a neurodiverse dyad (Strunz et al., 2017). This could be due to the greater understanding of each other's needs and, in particular, less emotional demands on each other and respect for the others' need for space and time to dedicate to their interests and hobbies. For example, an autistic couple who had shared their lives together for over 25 years both had interests that involved collecting. For one it was fishing magazines and for the other it was empty perfume bottles. Over the years their collections had become quite extensive and took over the majority of two rooms. Both showed total respect for each other's collections and never moved the items or suggested that either should discard any of their collections.

INTUITIVE UNDERSTANDING OF A PARTNER

It is becoming quite evident that it is difficult for autistic and non-autistic partners to intuitively understand each other. It was initially believed that the majority of misunderstandings were due to the autistic individual's difficulty reading non-verbal body language, automatically picking up social cues, and correctly interpreting voice tones and emphasis. Research is now discovering that this works in two ways and that it is also likely that non-autistic individuals have similar problems when trying to read autistic individuals (the double empathy problem).

Due to a lack of subtle facial expressions and eye contact at key points in the conversation, autistic individuals can be very difficult to read, and this can cause misunderstandings of their true intentions. Finding someone difficult to read has been connected to being perceived disapprovingly (Anders et al., 2016), and this can come at a great cost to autistic individuals when in a relationship with a non-autistic partner. To state a few examples: giving inappropriate signals, such as evasive eye contact, can easily be interpreted as being dishonest or embarrassed; smiling when the partner is distressed can be interpreted as being uncaring or even callous; making a joke about a sensitive subject can appear as cruel or indifferent; making too much eye contact can be seen as flirting or being aggressive, to name but a few. The chances of being misread and misunderstood are high for an autistic individual when communicating with non-autistic individuals. This is greatly increased if there is no awareness or understanding of autism by their partner or relationship counsellor.

Trying to fit into the non-autistic world requires masking and this can come at a great cost as described in the following quote taken from a study by Crompton, Hallet et al. (2020, p. 1443, Participant 3):

> After spending time with neurotypical friends, I feel wiped out, completely exhausted. I need to lie in a darkened room for 3–4 hours and when I do, I don't sleep, I just shut off. I can't even move and the only way I can communicate is in humming noises.

Feeling exhausted after a social event is often the reality for autistic individuals, but this will not always fit in with the dynamics of a couple's relationship, especially if one partner lacks a thorough understanding of autism. It is unlikely the non-autistic partner would understand why, when they return home from a visit to a family gathering, their autistic partner will not communicate and just want to lie down alone, especially when, for example, there are children to attend to and put to bed. Both partners will feel uncared for, both will feel unfairly misunderstood, and both will feel their needs are not being heard or met.

Partner responsiveness was the key predictor of relationship satisfaction that was found in a study of autistic and non-autistic individuals in a long-term neurodiverse relationship (Yew et al., 2023). This important finding highlights the importance of showing a partner that they are cared for, supported and validated. All the participants in this study were aware that they were in an autistic neurodiverse relationship, which also highlights the importance of being aware and understanding what that means for them. It is important for a counsellor to be aware that when working with a neurodiverse couple, it is unlikely that both partners will bring to counselling a shared experience of how they are feeling and managing within the relationship. The autistic partner is liable to hold a very different perspective and quite a different set of needs to those expressed by the non-autistic partner.

Relationship counselling should seek to educate both partners on each other's needs so that they can support, validate and offer the care that their partner requires to maintain a healthy level of relationship satisfaction.

THE REALITY OF THE RELATIONSHIP

Although the desire to form an intimate relationship can be quite strong for the autistic individual, sometimes the reality of what it actually means in terms of the cost to their routines and freedom to spend unlimited time with their interests is overlooked. Restrictions and new responsibilities can come as quite a shock when it is realized that this freedom is no longer practical or achievable without causing their partner to react unfavourably. Having time to spend on their chosen interests and being able to incorporate order and routines into their daily life are all essential requirements for most autistic individuals. If these are overly restricted or disallowed, they are likely to negatively impact the autistic individual's ability to maintain good mental health and well-being. In light of this, the autistic partner will endeavour, at all costs, to find the time for their interests and incorporate daily routines into the family life.

If neither partner is aware their relationship is neurodiverse, both will believe that their reality is the correct one and it is their partner who has the problem. Due to the lack of partner responsiveness shown to them, the non-autistic partner may eventually become less communicative and give up trying to discuss their feelings. This silence may go unheeded by an autistic partner, who will be totally unaware that something is wrong and will continue to focus on their interests and their own needs. Unfortunately, this behaviour could be misunderstood and perceived as unloving and uncaring by the non-autistic partner. This imbalance in the relationship cannot be maintained and will inevitably reach a critical point. This is when the autistic partner may find themselves having to make a choice between couple counselling or facing a separation.

This can come as quite a surprise for the autistic partner, as the signs that their partner was so unhappy and that their behaviour was the reason for this may have been totally overlooked. This is often due to the fact it was never their intention to cause their partner to be unhappy or to want to end the relationship. It is simply due to not understanding how it felt for their partner. This is shown clearly in the example below:

> I wasn't aware. I had situations where I would be sitting on a chair, she would be on the floor bawling her eyes out and say, 'why can't you understand?' And I would say 'understand what?' (Wilson et al., 2017, p. 8)

Both partners are likely to feel the victim in this scenario because neither understands the differences that exist between them and just how diverse their requirements from each other are. Their opposing needs in the relationship to maintain emotional and mental well-being will unavoidably be in conflict if not understood. Relationship counselling will need to address this and offer an authentic understanding of the conflicting scenario that will unfold before them in the counselling room.

It is important that the counsellor can offer each partner the education and support they need to develop a healthy comprehension of each other's reality. The counsellor will need to be clear and logical when explaining to the autistic partner the reasons behind their partner's unhappiness and what they can do about it. This will require patience as the information given may, for the autistic partner, take longer to process, comprehend and apply within the relationship.

EMPATHY

Autistic individuals experience empathy, but when responding to another's emotions it is unlikely to be spontaneous. The autistic partner will need the situation explained clearly in a way that they can understand. That might be by using analogies or metaphors that relate to their interests or by using colours, numbers or a visual means that is appropriate. Sometimes, it requires just stating the obvious, such as saying, 'If your partner cries it is okay to ask if she wants a hug'. Once the autistic partner understands what is required of them and knows it is safe to act on the advice, they are more likely to respond as expected and needed by their partner.

SENSORY SENSITIVITY

An area that can come at a great cost to the autistic partner when in a neurodiverse relationship is one which is not always obvious or discussed openly, and that is issues over sensory sensitivity. We have both witnessed times when disclosures regarding sensory issues by the autistic partner are only first revealed in counselling. These issues may have been ongoing for years but were not addressed as the autistic partner did not feel confident enough to bring them up or doubted their partner would understand and provide compassion for their sensory experiences. The reasons behind the non-disclosure can be due to the realization, gained at an early age, that other children did not react in the same way. While they found it highly stressful managing a specific noise, smell or being touched, their classmates were not affected in the same way and seemed to manage their sensory reactions well. Consequently, the autistic child learns quickly to mask their sensory reactions and find alternative ways of managing the effect.

Avoidance is often the primary method used to manage aversive sensory experiences, and that might mean avoiding noisy environments, eating with the family, avoiding participating in childcare routines or sleeping with their partner. Unfortunately, the outcome of this is that the non-autistic partner will interpret this avoidance behaviour as not wanting to share events, childcare, family life or intimacy with them. They will see this behaviour as not caring for or loving them and this will have an adverse negative effect on the relationship.

When the true reason for the autistic partner's behaviour is disclosed and understood by the non-autistic partner, strategies can be implemented, and the personal element can be removed. This will make for a more harmonious relationship for both partners. However, it will not take away the daily struggle with sensory sensitivity that the autistic partner will need to manage.

It will be important for relationship counselling to initiate exploration into this area, rather than waiting for the issues to be raised by the couple, by making use of the Sensory Sensitivity Questionnaire (Aston, 2021, pp. 120–124). This can be extended to suit the individual autistic partner the counsellor is working with. Sensory sensitivity can branch out into many areas, some of which are less obvious than others. Sometimes it can be just specific situations or a singular aspect of a situation. For example, if the issue that causes a negative reaction for the autistic partner is the noise caused by eating and chewing food, it could be presumed that this applies to all noise caused by eating food. However, this is rarely the case, and it may only be eating an apple or munching crisps and popcorn. The eating of other foods may not be an issue. Further exploration of this may then discover that the rustling noise of the bag that contains the crisps and popcorn is the cause of the main irritation factor. So, when they were replaced in a plastic bag, the reaction was dampened. The couple can be encouraged to explore aversive sensory experiences in some detail to be more precise in determining the specific trigger for the extreme distress.

Some reactions to sensory experiences can be interpreted as simply quirky and will just be laughed away or ignored, such as jumping when a sudden noise is heard, or not wanting to use hand dryers in public toilets. Equally, the individual might be hyposensitive and able to pick up hot plates or have a filling without a pain relief injection. These individual reactions will not impact the relationship or cause friction between the couple. However, environmental issues may still be causing stress and anxiety to the autistic partner and will be using up valuable cognitive resources required to get them through their daily lives and avoid meltdowns.

MELTDOWNS

Meltdowns can take three different forms: fight, flight or freeze, none of which are pleasant. For the majority of autistic adults, we have found that the flight and freeze reactions are the most usual, as the individual will have learnt to replace the fight response that can display itself in childhood and adolescence with the less interpersonally damaging flight or freeze. If, however, in relationship counselling the autistic partner is reacting with the fight response then this will need to be addressed.

A fight response can feel quite threatening to those around; it can take the form of shouting, abusive language, breaking objects and making threats, and sometimes it is turned inwards, and harm is caused to oneself. There is a release of powerful energy that can be destructive in terms of objects or aggression towards a person. We would recommend that the autistic partner be referred to individual counselling to work on changing this response so that harm to others and self can be avoided. We would like to add here that if the relationship is affected by domestic abuse, regardless of who is the abusive partner, then the counsellor should deal with this in accordance with their ethical or organizational guidelines. Autism cannot be used as an excuse for any form of domestic abuse and does not take away legal responsibility for this very unacceptable behaviour.

Meltdowns are one area that most autistic individuals will try their best to avoid, as this can mean losing control and being in a place that they do not want to be. Witnessing a 'fight response' meltdown by a partner or their family can be very distressing and disturbing, unlike the flight or freeze response, which, although it can arouse feelings of abandonment and frustration, is less damaging to others in the long term.

The autistic partner will likely have learnt strategies and coping skills to help them avoid becoming overwhelmed and experiencing a meltdown. For some, this may be using a distraction such as their interest or playing music; for others, it may be using mindfulness or going to the gym or for a run as a constructive release of energy. All these will be ways of self-soothing, which plays a valuable role in maintaining healthy mental and physical well-being.

These self-soothing techniques should be encouraged and never prevented. However, this may not be possible to maintain within a hectic family life and the constraints caused by being in a relationship. Relationship counselling will need to explore and discover what self-soothing techniques are used by the autistic partner. Look for ways that they can be beneficially modified, strengthened and maintained. Put together ways for both partners to be aware if a meltdown is developing and how it can be managed and prevented if possible. This will require the cooperation of both partners, and both will greatly benefit from incorporating self-soothing techniques into their daily couple lives.

ADVANTAGES OF HAVING AN AUTISTIC PARTNER

We have discussed the major challenges for the autistic individual of being in a neurodiverse relationship. These have included being misunderstood, time restrictions to spend on one's own interests, sensory sensitivity and meltdowns. Some of these can be quite debilitating for the autistic partner; they do not, however, appear to prevent most autistic individuals from forming relationships, and these relationships appear to be mainly with non-autistic partners. Despite the many challenges faced by autistic individuals when entering into a neurodiverse relationship there are also many advantages.

Research is now discovering the benefits for autistic individuals of being in the company of other autistic individuals (Crompton, Ropar et al., 2020) and that in autistic relationships the ratings were higher on relationship satisfaction scores than when in neurodiverse relationships (Strunz et al., 2017). It cannot be said however that autistic dyads do not also experience difficulties, as was found by Holmes (2023) who received negative reports from two autistic couples declaring their relationship was made very complicated and challenging due to the competing sensory profiles experienced by them.

MOTIVATION TO EXPERIENCE A LONG-TERM RELATIONSHIP

Many factors influence partner choice in forming an intimate relationship, including physical attraction, shared interests and values, personality, locality to each other, financial status and many more. These factors apply to all individuals. Our work has shown us just how motivated autistic adults are and how much effort they will make to initiate and form a romantic relationship. We have both spent time teaching relationship skills and supporting young autistic adults in finding a relationship and supporting them through the minefield of dating and courtship.

RELATIONSHIP SATISFACTION

The majority of relationships that we have worked with have been long term and resulted in a family. The majority have also been neurodiverse rather than autistic couplings. Research has found that in a neurodiverse dyad, it is more likely to be the non-autistic partner that reports a lower satisfaction with the relationship than the autistic partner (Strunz et al., 2017). This has been backed by reports we have both heard from the many neurodiverse couples we have supported over the years. The majority of dissatisfaction in the relationship has been voiced by the non-autistic partner rather than the autistic partner. The reasons for this are discussed in Chapter 11.

Despite the many challenges autistic partners have faced to be in a relationship, they have reported a decrease in the feelings of loneliness they were experiencing prior to the relationship. They have reported they felt more accepted within society and had their physical needs met, whether that be their partner dealing with the weekly shopping or cooking healthy meals. Most importantly, they felt they had someone they could rely on to be their social guide and deal with their social commitments and arrangements, whether that be connected to their work or personal life. One autistic gentleman who worked as a GP within a village community explained how his non-autistic partner dealt with all the telephone calls and any general concerns and queries. She was basically his social receptionist, and he relied on her communication and social skills to support him in his role as a GP.

Most essential for many autistic individuals is that their partner may be their only form of emotional support and will be a vital and valuable addition in their lives. This can be a benefit that very much outweighs the challenges that a neurodiverse relationship presents for them. Perhaps the biggest challenge for autistic individuals is knowing how to keep their partner happy and putting this into practice long term, which brings us to our next chapter, exploring 'What the autistic partner needs from relationship counselling'.

REFERENCES

Anders, S., de Jong, R., Beck, C., Haynes, J., & Ethofer, T. T. (2016). A neural link between affective understanding and interpersonal attraction. *Proceedings of the National Academy of Sciences of the United States of America, 113*, 2248–2257. https://doi.org/10.1073/pnas.1516191113

Aston, M. (2021). *The autism couple's workbook*. Jessica Kingsley Publishers.

Crompton, C. J., Hallett, S., Ropar, D., Flynn, E., & Fletcher-Watson, S. (2020). 'I never realised everybody felt as happy as I do when I am around autistic people': A thematic analysis of autistic adults' relationships with autistic and neurotypical friends and family. *Autism, 24*(6), 1438–1448. https://doi.org/10.1177/1362361320908976

Crompton, C. J., Ropar, D., Evans-Williams, C. V., Flynn, E. G., & Fletcher-Watson, S. (2020). Autistic peer-to-peer information transfer is highly effective. *Autism, 24*(7), 1704–1712. https://doi.org/10.1177/1362361320919286

Holmes, S. (2023). Exploring a later-in-life diagnosis and its impact on marital satisfaction in the lost generation of autistic adults: An exploratory phenomenological qualitative study. *Global Journal of Intellectual & Developmental Disabilities, 12*. https://doi.org/10.19080/GJIDD.2023.12.555829

Strunz, S., Schermuck, C., Ballerstein, S., Ahlers, C. J., Dziobek, I., & Roepke, S. (2017). Romantic relationships and relationship satisfaction among adults with Asperger syndrome and high-functioning autism. *Journal of Clinical Psychology, 73*(1), 113–125. https://doi.org/10.1002/jclp.22319

Wilson, B., Beamish, W., Hay, S., & Attwood, T. (2017). The communication 'roundabout': Intimate relationships of adults with Asperger syndrome. *Cogent Psychology, 4*(1), 1283828. https://doi.org/10.1080/23311908.2017.1283828

Yew, R. Y., Hooley, M., & Stokes, M. (2023). Factors of relationship satisfaction for autistic and non-autistic partners in long-term relationships. *Autism, 27*(8). https://doi.org/10.1177/13623613231160244

What the Autistic Partner Needs from Relationship Counselling

It is quite clear from research and the respondents in our survey that when most autistic individuals commit to a relationship, they are there for the long haul. Research has found that rather than seeking short-term relationships, autistic individuals show a much stronger desire and commitment towards long-term and monogamous relationships. This was backed up by our survey, which found the average length of relationships was 20 years, and the longest was 50 years. Within the 225 respondents infidelity was not raised once as an issue within the relationship. These findings are unique considering it is estimated that one in five adults will have an affair, and should come as a major plus for anyone in a relationship with an autistic partner. Infidelity is stated to be responsible for 20 to 40% of divorces in the USA.

The majority of autistic partners we have worked with who are in a relationship would not consider having an affair and are intensely loyal to their partners. Equally, they are often, but not always, hardworking and conscientious and seek to be in a position to provide for their partner and family. So why are their non-autistic partners not content and satisfied and feel the need for them both to attend relationship counselling?

The answer to this is that despite the qualities that the autistic partner offers, they are not always very adept at showing their partner that they love and care for them. There can be a tendency for the autistic partner to become totally absorbed in their own world, especially their hobbies and interests, thus becoming perceived as unresponsive to their partner's needs and emotions. Although the non-autistic partner will have been showing their unhappiness and voicing their concerns, these indicators can be misread and overlooked by the autistic partner, especially if they are unaware that they are a neurodiverse couple. This oversight is not intentional; it is due to the difficulties posed in reading their partner's non-verbal body language and interpreting their intentions accurately. The autistic partner may feel that their partner is being irrational, overemotional and unfairly critical, failing to understand that they are being unresponsive to their partner's genuine need to be emotionally supported and feel cared for. The reality of this need will often not be addressed by the autistic partner and may add to lengthening the distance that is developing between them.

It can feel for the autistic partner that the only problem with their relationship is their partner, who whatever they do never seems to be satisfied. This probably explains why the autistic client will often appear in the counselling room as being quite mystified and confused as to what it is that is going so wrong in their relationship and why their partner is so unhappy and critical of them. There will be feelings expressed of not being understood, which can often result in the autistic partner feeling like a failure in the relationship.

FEELING UNDERSTOOD BY THE RELATIONSHIP COUNSELLOR

The autistic partner will need to feel understood by the relationship counsellor and will pick up very quickly if this is not immediately apparent. Our survey showed that lack of understanding from the counsellor was named as one of the main causes of counselling failure, regardless of whether the relationship counsellor had advertised as being knowledgeable in this area.

It will be impossible to establish trust, security and safety within the therapeutic relationship if a genuine understanding is not offered by the counsellor. Without understanding autism, inappropriate exercises and strategies were shown to be suggested by the relationship counsellor in our survey. This had a very negative effect on the couple's relationship and further enhanced the autistic partner's feelings of being misunderstood, causing much damage to their self-esteem and confidence in the therapeutic process. Once understanding and trust are established, the autistic partner will feel able to voice their needs safely and to be able to ask some very pertinent questions. This will be in the hope that the relationship counsellor can provide the answers they need.

Below, we have listed some of the most common questions asked of the relationship counsellor.

TELL ME HOW I CAN MAKE MY PARTNER HAPPY

This is the question that we have been asked so many times by autistic partners, who are often quite confused as to why their partner is so unhappy. As an autistic gentleman stated, 'I work hard, I pay all the bills, I taxi the children around, I do jobs for her around the house and still she complains that she feels neglected!'.

We hear of how baffled the autistic partner is often left feeling. Unfortunately, they have no idea what their partner is expecting them to do or say. Consequently, over time, they will have learnt to just withdraw when a situation becomes emotional, as it is difficult to try to resolve a problem when you don't know what the problem is.

Relationship counselling will need to address the importance of the autistic partner understanding what their non-autistic partner needs from them and why. This will require being logical and clear and highlighting the distinction between meeting their partner's practical needs and meeting their emotional needs. Referring to *The Five Languages of Love That Lasts* (Chapman, 2015) can offer good reading and validation of how important it is to be aware of the differing needs that exist between partners.

The counsellor could help the non-autistic partner to put together a list of ways (that do not rely on emotional dialogue) that the autistic partner might be able to meet some of their non-autistic partner's needs. It is important that the list is kept as practical and logical as possible, avoiding the need for the autistic partner to participate in conversations and discussions centred on their emotions. This list will be very individual to the partner compiling it and may include various ideas, such as 'holding my hand when we go for a walk', 'sitting by me when we watch a film together', 'giving me a hug when I ask for one'. Having a list of requirements and instructions can come as a great relief for the autistic partner, and most will do their best to fulfil it and maybe more. Buying an occasional card expressing love and appreciation and writing I love you can be a very effective way of meeting a non-autistic partner's emotional needs.

Relationship counselling will require educating and working with both partners to achieve a balance within the relationship, and both helping the autistic partner find a way to show they care and teaching the non-autistic partner that love can take many forms, and helping both to understand the love languages of their partner.

I JUST CAN'T WIN: WHATEVER I SAY IT IS WRONG AND IF I DON'T SAY ANYTHING THAT IS WRONG TOO. WHY?

Over time, a history of misunderstandings can build up between the couple, and, along with many failed attempts to find a resolution, this can result in the couple ceasing to communicate and distancing themselves emotionally. This scenario takes time to develop, and often the initial reaction from the autistic partner is one of distress. When the misunderstandings continue, distress may be replaced by defensiveness and depression. Unfortunately, the outcome of this will be a withdrawal by both partners accompanied by a total breakdown in any attempt to converse.

In the first instance, the autistic partner is likely to become quite distressed to realize that they have given the wrong answer or reaction, often declaring or promising to their partner that they will not do it again. It is, though, likely that this will be without understanding what it is they are not going to do again. Due to this, it is likely that the scenario will be repeated, and they will be met with even more dissatisfaction from their partner. Their non-autistic partner will not be aware of why this has happened again and feel let down and insecure in the autistic partner's ability to keep their word.

Next time this occurs, the autistic partner is more likely to become defensive before their partner even has the chance to voice their discontent, which could result in an expression of anger and frustration. Finally, the autistic partner will learn that it is easier to walk away and not get involved in an argument as they will feel that they are being attacked by their partner and that their partner is being overemotional. It is likely that by now, as they still are not aware of what they are not doing right, they will be blaming the non-autistic partner for the misunderstandings and arguments so will be more likely to withdraw (Wilson et al., 2017).

Relationship counselling will need to explain to the autistic partner that withdrawing and walking away will only exacerbate the rift and problems that exist between the couple. The non-autistic partner will need to be aware that unless an agreement is made to listen without interrupting and it feels safe for the autistic partner to discuss together an issue, then it is unlikely any attempt to achieve this will happen. It can be very difficult for the non-autistic partner to suppress feelings of hurt and frustration, as these may have been building up over many years. We would advise that initially, the counsellor recommends that the couple bring any unresolved areas of conflict to the counselling room to discuss these only with a third party present.

The counsellor's role will then be one of translator and sometimes referee. Some issues cannot be resolved, and the counsellor will be hearing two perceptions that are so far apart it will be difficult to believe that the couple were both present at the same time. If this occurs, we suggest that it would be unachievable to try to knit together the differing perspectives and find a way of agreeing to disagree and let the matter go.

Explain to both partners that neither perception is wrong because perception is subjective, and each should be addressed and given credence by the counsellor. The counsellor will need to show that they empathize with each partner and understand how difficult it is for them. It can be almost impossible to rectify issues from the past as it is not possible to change or alter what has already happened. Counselling can, though, teach the couple how to deal with issues as they occur in the present, working with the couple to develop and form strategies to help them manage any issues that arise. Recommend to the autistic client that rather than walk away and stay silent, they should go to another room and write down their thoughts in an email or text message, and their partner, in return, should answer in the same way. This will avoid the difficulties caused by misreading facial expressions, tone of voice and gestures which indicate each other's thoughts and intentions.

WHY DO I FIND IT SO HARD TO CONVERSE WITH MY FAMILY/ PARTNER WHEN I COME HOME? I JUST WANT TO BE ON MY OWN

For the autistic partner, it can be difficult to make a spontaneous transition from work to home life, and an amount of time will be needed to mentally process the change of structure, environment and expectations. This is perfectly normal for an autistic individual and is something that should be built into the relationship and become part of the family routine.

If the couple were not aware they were neurodiverse or as yet do not understand what it means, then relationship counselling will need to educate both on the relevance of processing time and the need for a calming and energy-restoring transition between work and home.

Both partners in a neurodiverse relationship will have different needs and require different strategies to keep themselves mentally and physically healthy. For the non-autistic partner, this will mean talking about their day with their partner and family. This is in direct contrast with the needs of the autistic partner, who may require some time to internally process their day, may not see any personal value in disclosing the day's events to their partner and will find solace and energy restoration in their solitary hobbies and interests.

For one autistic partner, their way of winding down was to arrive home and put on a quiz show, becoming totally absorbed in answering the questions. This was not appreciated by their partner, who was eager for them to discuss their day together and get on with the household chores. A compromise was to limit the time that the autistic partner could spend alone, to say 30 minutes, and then to join the family in the kitchen to allow the non-autistic partner to discuss their day, and this was also limited to 30 minutes. This soon became a pattern and sufficed as meeting both sets of needs in the family.

A relationship counsellor will need to explore the needs of each couple they work with, as needs will be individual and require a different working compromise. Whatever is decided, it is essential that the autistic partner is allowed the time and space to make the transition from work to home and to process their thoughts and the day's events. Allowing this will benefit all the family.

WHY DO I FEEL MY PARTNER MISUNDERSTANDS EVERYTHING I SAY?

Feeling understood by one's partner is shown to have a very positive effect on couple relationships (Oishi et al., 2008). Feeling constantly misunderstood is going to have the opposite effect. Reports from both partners struggling with communication are frequently voiced in relationship counselling. Both partners will be trying to get their point across, and relationship counselling will need to explain that the feelings they both express of not being understood are very common in neurodiverse relationships. Misunderstandings in communication occur because both are, without realizing it, talking in a different 'language' and from a different perspective. The counsellor will need to reassure both and offer explanations as to why this keeps happening.

Much time in relationship counselling will be spent translating between the couple and teaching each how to communicate in a way that the other can understand. Some couples will be able to devise ways that work well for them. For others, already exhausted from attempts to remedy this, they may need time and patience to build up their energy levels before they can try again.

Relationship counselling should focus on conflict resolution and encouraging positive communication between the couple, taking time to explore every avenue possible to improve communication and enable the couple to avoid conflict caused by misunderstandings.

WHY IS MY PARTNER ANGRY ALL THE TIME WITH ME?

We have found that as well as misreading the non-autistic partner's facial expressions and voice tone, there is also a strong likelihood that whatever their expression it will more likely be interpreted as negative than positive by the autistic partner. When applying the 'Mind in the Eyes' test (Baron-Cohen et al., 2001) to autistic individuals, we have found that negative emotions are chosen far more frequently by the autistic individual than positive emotions. For example, out of four choices autistic individuals often chose the label 'irritable' to describe the emotion eyes in a picture were showing when, in fact, an 'irritable' expression was not included in the test. When an autistic partner has difficulty determining the emotion conveyed in their partner's facial expressions, there can be an automatic assumption that the emotion being conveyed is anger, and they respond accordingly.

Using this test can be a very helpful way of illustrating to the autistic partner that they are misreading emotions, and are likely to be misreading their partner too. In addition, this illustrates well to the non-autistic partner that they are being misread and need to clarify that their partner has understood the intentions behind their communication, whether verbal or non-verbal.

Relationship counselling will need to explain this to the autistic partner and can, with the couple's consent, use this very informative test to clearly illustrate what is occurring between them. The test is easily accessible online.

WHY IS IT SUCH A BIG DEAL FOR MY PARTNER/FAMILY TO MANAGE TO BE READY ON TIME? WE ARE ALWAYS LATE

A need for promptness or to arrive early can be very important for the autistic partner and if the family are like-minded this will not present as an issue in the relationship. This adherence to time does not affect all autistic individuals and, for some, due to executive functioning difficulties, the opposite can be true and getting somewhere on time can be the issue.

The driver here is anxiety; it is often the fear of the unexpected occurring that causes much anxiety for autistic individuals. Maintaining control and avoiding unforeseen circumstances taking over can be paramount in reducing anxiety and avoiding situations that could become overwhelming and produce a meltdown. Leaving early means any unforeseen delays can more easily be accommodated and not being criticized for being late.

Relationship counselling will need to help find strategies and teach ways for the autistic partner to de-stress and find some calm within these situations. Going for a brief walk or finding a distraction while the family are getting ready can help. Encourage the non-autistic partner not to give a precise time that they will be ready by; for example, rather than say, 'I will be a couple of minutes', when that deadline is not achievable, say, I will be ready in between 10 and 20 minutes. If possible, delegate a job for the autistic partner to be doing while everyone is getting ready, for example loading up the car or taking the dog for a quick walk. Anything that creates a useful distraction will help keep anxiety levels low and create a feeling of being in control.

BIRTHDAYS, CHRISTMAS AND FAMILY REUNIONS SEEM SO IMPORTANT TO MY PARTNER, AND THEY COMPLAIN THAT I DON'T SHARE THEIR EXCITEMENT

Sharing joy for positive life events enhances relationship satisfaction (Gable et al., 2004). Relationship counselling will need to explain to the autistic partner how this is often the case for non-autistic individuals, and especially females.

These important social events, perhaps with many family members, can be overwhelming for an autistic partner. There is sudden laughter, perhaps balloons that could burst, being in close proximity to so many people and being expected to engage in small talk. There is a risk of social and sensory overload and thoughts are of endurance not excitement.

Giving and receiving presents are forms of emotional expression that tell the other they are cared for and loved. Taking the time to choose a gift or card, wrapping the gift, and writing the card are all reinforcers and affirmations of feeling loved and cared for. These positive reinforcers are, for some individuals, a vital component of the relationship and a way of achieving couple connectedness and a sense of belonging.

If this is something that is not being fulfilled by the autistic partner and is important to the non-autistic partner, then relationship counselling will need to explain that celebrating special events and making the effort to participate in exchanging gifts and cards will benefit both in the relationship.

The aim of the majority of autistic partners is to make their partner happy; however, how to achieve this is not always obvious. The counsellor will need to explore this and explain the benefits they will receive if they are willing to make the effort to attend and participate in such social gatherings. The counsellor will also need to explore other reasons that the autistic partner does not wish to participate, which can range from being in close proximity to relative strangers to personality clashes.

Another reason may be simply that special occasions were never celebrated by their childhood family and are therefore not relevant to them and/or they are unsure of anticipated family protocols and conventions. They may often presume that just because it is something they don't need or enjoy, then that also applies to their partner. This misassumption is something the counsellor will need to discuss with both partners.

Lack of participation can also be due to having tried and getting it wrong. Foolproof ways of avoiding this can be put into place by the non-autistic partner explaining the sequence of events, family etiquette, and compiling a list of appropriate gifts and potential topics of conversation with each participant (Aston, 2021). There are also advantages in highlighting forthcoming events on a calendar and phones, which will help prevent missing the date and being prepared.

We have found that once the autistic partner has a logical understanding of what is required of them and what they need to do, much effort can be made (Aston, 2012, p. 157).

MY PARTNER ACCUSES ME OF BEING OVERLY DEFENSIVE, BUT I FEEL THEY CONSTANTLY CRITICIZE ME AND EVERYTHING I DO OR SAY

A strong defensive reaction to any form of perceived criticism by the autistic partner is a problem that affects almost all autistic neurodiverse relationships. It can be what causes many of the failures in attempts by the couple to communicate and resolve any conflict between them.

Defensiveness is a reaction that is known to cause the downfall of many couple relationships in the population as a whole. Gottman (1999) identified it as the second of the four horsemen. The four horsemen were described as predictors of a divorce or a breakup between a couple. Defensiveness was described as a way to deny responsibility for the issue raised, which in turn only accelerates the conflict between the couple (Gottman, 1999).

Defensiveness in autistic individuals could possibly be due to the difficulty reading their partner's intentions, misreading their body language and often automatically assuming their partner is angry and on the attack. Very often, their partner is not attacking them, but when they are met with a highly defensive reaction, this will, as Gottman described, serve to turn the situation into one of conflict, which will in turn incorrectly confirm to the autistic partner that they were under attack.

Relationship counselling will need to break this destructive and self-defeating cycle that the couple may have got themselves into. This will not be easy to achieve and will only be resolved if the autistic partner can learn to realize that they are misreading their partner's intentions and not react defensively or for the non-autistic partner to not react to the defensive reaction. It may be easier to achieve the latter. If this cycle continues, it will inevitably lead to more distance between the couple and could result in an avoidance of communication altogether.

Once again how relationship counselling approaches this issue is dependent on the couple involved. The counsellor should work with the couple to list the positives in their partner and to show their appreciation for the attributes and strengths their partner brings to the relationship. Finding the positives will increase self-esteem and help to alleviate the feelings of failure that both might be experiencing.

WHY DO I KEEP GETTING ACCUSED OF FORGETTING SOMETHING I AM SURE WAS NEVER SAID?

If this is an issue in the relationship, then it could be due to a few reasons. The first and obvious explanation is that the autistic partner did not understand what it was their partner was trying to communicate to them. If something is not understood, then it is unlikely to find its way into long-term memory, much in the same way that if someone is talking in a different language, the message will not be understood and therefore not retained. The second reason why a message may be forgotten is that it was given at a time when the autistic partner was distracted, and they were not given enough time to focus their attention on the message that was being given. The third reason is that the important message was lost within too much other information or irrelevant details. A fourth reason is that the non-autistic partner was not clear in their communication and remembers what they thought they said rather than what they actually said. There will be times when one of these reasons is the cause and times when all four might be involved.

Relationship counselling will need to advise the non-autistic partner to only give one important message at a time and ask for the message to be repeated back to them to ensure comprehension and facilitate accurate recall. To enhance this, if the message is very important, then write it down or send it in an email or message and check for a reply.

The autistic partner will also need to make the effort to put reminders in their phone and not be afraid of asking their partner to repeat or explain what they have asked. The counsellor will need to teach the non-autistic partner the importance of giving messages at the right time, making them clear, writing instructions down and the need to be patient and repeat the request if asked.

MY PARTNER ACCUSES ME OF NOT BEING INTERESTED IN THEIR DAY. I DO NOT UNDERSTAND WHY, IF THEY HAVE SOMETHING IMPORTANT TO SAY, WHY CAN'T THEY JUST SAY IT?

Enquiring about a partner's day and how they are feeling all contribute towards feelings of belonging and being cared for. This type of partner inquiry, though, may not come naturally to the autistic partner who is often absorbed in their own day and thoughts. For many autistic partners there is confusion as to why their partner can't just tell them if they have something important to say. They express frustration at being expected to automatically know and for this to be a priority.

The non-autistic partner might have been giving lots of non-verbal hints that something is amiss and there is something they wish to share. Their expectation is that their partner should pick up on this and ask them how their day has been or if something is wrong. Due to difficulty in reading their partner's body language, the message may not have been picked up by the autistic partner. If they do have a sense that something is wrong, they are likely to assume it is because of something that they have done or not done and they are reluctant to know what, as this could lead to being criticized again. The consequence of this is that the autistic partner is likely to withdraw altogether rather than risk possible conflict. This behaviour will unfortunately exacerbate the situation.

Both perspectives make sense and are understandable when it is considered that the couple are neurodiverse and, therefore, not sharing the same needs and expectations of each other. Relationship counselling can educate the couple on these different needs as well as looking for a compromise. The simplest solution to this would be that the non-autistic partner did speak up and directly rather than indirectly say if there is something they wish to share. However, this solution will not alleviate their need to feel their partner is interested enough in them to inquire about their day or to ask them if there is anything they wish to talk about.

Various tools can be purchased online that clearly illustrate how someone is feeling and can be used and put in an obvious place for the autistic partner to see. For example, some couples have found that small pocket-sized books that illustrate an emoji facial expression on each page with the relevant emotion word printed underneath can be very useful for getting the message across, without having to verbally explain. Using the page with the word neglected and a sad face may be enough to inform the autistic partner that they need to inquire how their spouse is.

It is useful for the counsellor to have a supply of different tools on hand to allow the couple to practice and discover what works for them.

OUR PREVIOUS COUNSELLOR GAVE US EXERCISES THAT I COULDN'T DO, AND I ENDED UP FEELING LIKE A FAILURE

Reports from respondents in our research highlighted the difficulties the autistic partner faced when given exercises and tasks to complete that they were not realistically able to maintain. These tasks could include the couple taking turns to discuss their feelings with each other, or they might be asked to give each other a personal compliment every evening.

Tasks that require emotional expression, and especially spontaneous expression, can be very difficult for the autistic partner, and this is made less likely to be achieved if the autistic partner also experiences alexithymia.

Relationship counselling should avoid tasks that involve emotional expression and require the ability to figure out what the non-autistic partner wants to hear, without any direction, clarification or guidance. Worksheets that require using numbers, colour or completing question-naires should be employed. Example pages of handouts can be found in *The Autism Couple's Workbook* (Aston, 2021).

SHOULD I HAVE A DIAGNOSIS?

Getting a diagnosis is a very personal choice, and one that only the individual concerned should make. Relationship counselling should discuss the pros and cons of this choice in detail with the partner, considering whether they are autistic. We recommend this be done individually to allow uninhibited and open discussion of fears or concerns.

Research has found conflicting evidence regarding how beneficial a diagnosis is to a neurodiverse couple. Holmes (2023) found a higher marital dissatisfaction in neurodiverse couples when there was no aware-ness of autism or it was not diagnosed until after many years of being together. Of the 23 adults interviewed who had undergone an autism diagnosis, 11 reported it as positive and they felt it came as a relief to now be able to understand the differences between both partners. This was in contrast to three of the nine adults who saw the diagnosis as being negative declaring that it took away all hope for the non-autistic partner that anything in their relationship would change.

A study by Leedham et al. (2020) that explored the effects on women who received a diagnosis in later life found that, for the majority, the effects were beneficial. These benefits included being able to change their self-perception from being self-critical to self-compassionate. Participants also felt that a diagnosis gave them an understanding and an increased acceptance of themselves. Positive benefits to their relation-ships were also quoted as they felt more understood by their partners, as seen in the quotes below:

> ...he (husband) got really into researching it...it's really improved our relationship because he's realised that a lot of the arguments we had were me misunderstanding what he'd said and him misunderstanding how I'd reacted. (Leedham et al., 2020, p. 140)

> ...he'll (husband) now take the lead in situations where he knows I'm not comfortable, whereas before he just thought I was being awkward. (Leedham et al., 2020, p. 141)

Many participants in the study also reported that they experienced less distress and anxiety than they did before the diagnosis. A diagnosis did not solve all the difficulties the women experienced, but it did enable some major positive changes and allow for a much better understanding of self.

In the reports that we received from respondents, all described discovering autism and, for some, receiving a diagnosis to be very positive events in the relationship that helped remove the confusion and unrealistic expectations. Overall, the benefits of a diagnosis appear to outweigh the negatives, and it has been found to have a positive effect on the relationship (Jones et al., 2014: Parsloe, 2015; Smith et al., 2020). We also found this in our survey. A strong benefit for the autistic partner is permission to be themselves in the relationship and not having to camouflage their behaviour (Cage et al., 2018). However, this has been a downside for some non-autistic partners who expressed that their partner no longer made an effort to fit in or socialize.

Relationship counselling should look deeply into the reasons why the autistic individual wants a diagnosis, and we would recommend compiling a pros and cons chart together. Maybe use two different coloured pens for the pros and cons. The counsellor should encourage and prompt their client to give this much thought and to include the aspects of arranging an assessment, going for the assessment, who they would take with them and importantly how much it would cost, and waiting times if provided. There may be a consideration as to whether to seek out an assessment privately or try to find a way for this to be funded. Some individuals feel they would rather keep their diagnosis private and would prefer not to have it in their medical records; reasons for this can vary.

WHY IS IT SO IMPORTANT FOR MY PARTNER FOR ME TO HAVE A DIAGNOSIS? I WILL STILL BE ME

Sometimes, it can seem that confirmation of an autism diagnosis is more important for the non-autistic partner than it is for the autistic partner, and this is very understandable. Awareness of autism for some couples does not become apparent until they have been together for a longer period of time – some find out after decades of not knowing what it was that made them so different. The non-autistic partner may have spent years trying to figure out what was preventing both partners from being able to communicate and understand each other. A diagnosis will mean that friends, family and professionals will need to take their concerns seriously, and hopefully open up access to the appropriate support and strategies that both need to benefit their relationship. Discovering autism can feel like the answer to so many questions, and offer validation and a means of seeking support from other couples where one partner is autistic, reading literature on neurodiverse couples and not feeling so alone.

Unfortunately, we have both worked with couples where an ultimatum will be given by the non-autistic partner: 'You either get a diagnosis or I am leaving you'. This can result in the autistic partner feeling they do not really have a choice. Relationship counselling will need to address these conflicts and offer understanding to both partners. Being coerced into getting a diagnosis is not acceptable, and unfortunately a diagnosis does not come with any guarantee that it will make the relationship better. Fears that having a diagnosis will mean being blamed for everything going wrong have been often voiced in the counselling room by an autistic partner.

Acceptance of being autistic is far more important than having a formal diagnosis, and it is this acceptance, followed by the understanding of both partners, that offers the best chance of relationship survival. Relationship counselling will need to handle this scenario as sensitively as possible and educate both partners that simply being different is not the issue. It is not being aware of autism or not accepting the difference that will cause the main difficulties and barriers in achieving mutual relationship satisfaction.

REFERENCES

Aston, M. (2012). *What men with Asperger syndrome want to know about women, dating and relationships*. Jessica Kingsley Publishers.

Aston, M. (2021). *The autism couple's workbook* (2nd ed.). Jessica Kingsley Publishers.

Baron-Cohen, S., Wheelwright, S., Hill, J., Raste, Y., & Plumb, I. (2001). The 'Reading the Mind in the Eyes' Test revised version: A study with normal adults, and adults with Asperger syndrome or high-functioning autism. *Journal of Child Psychology and Psychiatry, 42*(2), 241–251. https://doi.org/10.1111/1469-7610.00715

Cage, E., Di Monaco, J., & Newell, V. (2018). Experiences of autism acceptance and mental health in autistic adults. *Journal of Autism and Developmental Disorders, 48*, 473–484. https://doi.org/10.1007/s10803-017-3342-7

Chapman, G. (2015). *The 5 love languages: The secret to love that lasts*. Northfield Publishing.

Gable, S. L., Reis, H. T., Impett, E. A., & Asher, E. R. (2004). What do you do when things go right? The intrapersonal and interpersonal benefits of sharing positive events.

Journal of Personality and Social Psychology, 87(2), 228–245. https://doi.org/10.1037/0022-3514.87.2.228

Gottman, J. M. (1999). *The marriage clinic: A scientifically based marital therapy.* W.W. Norton & Company.

Holmes, S. (2023). Exploring a later-in-life diagnosis and its impact on marital satisfaction in the lost generation of autistic adults: An exploratory phenomenological qualitative study. *Global Journal of Intellectual & Developmental Disabilities, 12.* https://doi.org/10.19080/GJIDD.2023.12.555829

Jones, L., Goddard, L., Hill, E. L., Henry, L., & Crane, L. (2014). Experiences of receiving a diagnosis of autism spectrum disorder: A survey of adults in the United Kingdom. *Journal of Autism and Developmental Disorders, 44*(12), 3033–3044. https://doi.org/10.1007/s10803-014-2161-3

Leedham, A., Thompson, A. R., Smith, R., & Freeth, M. (2020). 'I was exhausted trying to figure it out': The experiences of females receiving an autism diagnosis in middle to late adulthood. *Autism, 24*(1), 135–146. https://doi.org/10.1177/1362361319853442

Oishi, S., Koo, M., & Akimoto, S. (2008). Culture, interpersonal perceptions, and happiness in social interactions. *Personality and Social Psychology Bulletin, 34*(3), 307–320. https://doi.org/10.1177/0146167207311198

Parsloe, S. M. (2015). Discourses of disability, narratives of community: Reclaiming an autistic identity online. *Journal of Applied Communication Research, 43*(3), 336–356. https://doi.org/10.1080/00909882.2015.1052829

Smith, R., Netto, J., Gribble, N., & Falkmer, M. (2020). 'At the end of the day, it's love': An exploration of relationships in neurodiverse couples. *Journal of Autism and Developmental Disorders, 51*(9), 3311–3321. https://doi.org/10.1007/s10803-020-04790-z

Wilson, B., Beamish, W., Hay, S., & Attwood, T. (2017). The communication 'roundabout': Intimate relationships of adults with Asperger syndrome. *Cogent Psychology, 4*(1), 1283828. https://doi.org/10.1080/23311908.2017.1283828

CHAPTER 14

The Autistic Female Partner in a Relationship

Autistic women, much like their male counterparts, exhibit the same core autistic traits. However, they are often expected to conform to societal norms of femininity, such as gentleness, empathy, humility and sensitivity. This expectation can present gender-based hurdles for autistic women in establishing and sustaining relationships. Autistic women may have consciously adopted the accepted social construct of femininity or grappled with being accepted as their authentic selves, thereby adding another layer of complexity to their relationship dynamics. Their resilience in navigating these societal expectations is truly commendable.

Traditionally, our understanding of autism has been heavily skewed towards males, with a presumed gender ratio of 4:1. This bias is evident in research studies and relationship support literature, which predominantly feature the male partner as the autistic individual. However, recent findings have challenged this perspective, revealing a gender ratio of 2:1 male to female among autistic adults (Posserud et al., 2021). This shift in understanding is a significant step towards comprehending the experiences of autistic women in relationships. However, our current understanding is primarily derived from counselling experiences rather than extensive research data.

HISTORY OF FRIENDSHIPS FOR AUTISTIC WOMEN

Childhood and adolescent friendships are a foundation stone for adult relationships. A study of current and former friendships and romantic relationships of autistic women aged 20–40 found that autistic women have fewer, more intense friendships than their non-autistic peers (Sedgewick et al., 2019). The degree of intensity has sometimes resulted in friends disengaging. The autistic research participants tended to lack a wide social network, with an individual best friend often being the sole focus of their social lives. However, there was greater friendship satisfaction and stability in the mature years.

During the adolescent years, autistic teenage girls are vulnerable to relational bullying, such as being the focus of gossip, derogatory comments and being deliberately excluded from friendship groups. A compensation strategy for these experiences can be to consciously suppress autistic characteristics and analyse and imitate the social interactions of their peers. We use the terms camouflaging or masking, and research has found that autistic women are more likely to take on masking behaviours than autistic men (Lai et al., 2017). Another compensation strategy is for autistic girls and women to seek and enjoy the company of males since their social dynamics are relatively simpler and less rejecting, and they accept a 'tomboy' in their group. Thus, their friendship experiences have been unconventional compared to non-autistic female peers, emphasizing suppressing the authentic self and 'acting' in social situations to gain social acceptance or not developing the conventional same-gender friendships and conventional female persona.

HISTORY OF RELATIONSHIPS

Unfortunately, due to delayed Theory of Mind abilities, autistic adults can have difficulty determining the thoughts, feelings and intentions of others. They may not perceive the warning signals to identify malicious intentions intuitively. We have found that many autistic women have experienced abuse in friendships and relationships and often describe unwanted sexual experiences. This can be due to naivety, especially misinterpreting intentions and low self-esteem.

Research by Gibbs et al. (2021) used a cross-sectional survey of autistic and non-autistic adults (male and female). The authors of the study noted that 46% of autistic women reported having experienced sexual violence compared to 17% of autistic men. They also found that autistic adults are more likely to report that they had never confided to anyone about experiencing sexual violence. As trust develops in a relationship, an autistic woman may eventually feel confident disclosing such traumatic experiences to their partner or disclosing them for the first time to a relationship counsellor.

A study by Pecora et al. (2020) found that autistic women had an interest in romantic relationships as much as non-autistic women but had less social insight, greater social victimization and difficulties initiating and establishing relationships. There were also difficulties in achieving sexual knowledge from peers, and some perceived engagement in sexual behaviour as a means of attaining social approval from peers and facilitating a relationship experience. Participants in the research study also described how they were often unaware they were being taken advantage of.

AN ABUSIVE RELATIONSHIP

Some autistic women may exhibit low self-esteem and fear of rejection. They may have no close friends to provide advice on their prospective partner's intentions and reputation. As an autistic woman explained, 'I set my expectations very low and, as a result, gravitated toward abusive people. I cannot stress enough the importance of recognizing how important self-esteem is to an autistic adult'. Another autistic woman explained, 'We have good radar but talk ourselves out of it'. An autistic woman's compassion for her abusive partner can maintain the relationship, as described in the following quotation from our counselling experience: 'Got to give them a chance, not to make rash judgements, we don't want to treat people badly. Need to give them the benefit of the doubt'. The abuse can include verbal, emotional, physical, sexual and financial abuse.

We have also found that autistic women often struggled to know how to leave a potentially abusive relationship and were likely to stay in the relationship because that was easier than finding a new one. However, they might initiate a referral to a relationship counsellor.

Working with a client who is in an abusive relationship can prove challenging for a counsellor, especially if the abuse is not being recognized or accepted by the client. The counsellor will need to thoroughly assess the situation as it will be important to follow the recommended guidelines of their professional body.

If abuse is found to exist in any couple relationship the counsellor should not work with the couple together, as this could serve to exacerbate the situation. The abusive partner would need to be referred to a perpetrator programme or for specialized counselling. If there are children involved then immediate measures should be taken to ensure their safety. The case should be discussed with a supervisor and then the guidelines recommended for safeguarding issues should be followed.

CURRENT RELATIONSHIP ISSUES

We have noted that autistic women can have talents in the creative arts, have a deep empathic connection with animals, provide practical help and advice, and be open and honest, often with a strong sense of social justice. They may also have a successful career in the caring professions. A prospective partner can appreciate all of these characteristics.

One of the camouflaging characteristics of autistic women is noticing that non-autistic women often initiate a conversation with another woman by complimenting their conversation partner's fashionable clothing, hairstyle and makeup. An autistic woman may develop expertise in being fashionable to engage with other women socially. Men would also find this characteristic attractive when first meeting their autistic partner. As an autistic woman camouflages her autism, she may personify the ideal female partner. Eventually, the hope is that her partner sees and loves the authentic self rather than the mask. If not, a deep disappointment may be expressed in relationship counselling.

Autism is associated with having intense interests, and autistic adolescent girls can develop an intense interest in a person as a 'crush', and in their adult years, the 'crush' could be a prospective partner. As one autistic woman said, 'My husband essentially became my special interest'. In the early stages of the relationship, there may be aspects that resemble stalking and infatuation. The intensity of adulation can end the relationship or intoxicate both partners. One of the characteristics of special interests is that there is a 'use by date', meaning the initial intensity will over time be replaced by indifference, which may be a theme for relationship counselling.

Conventional wisdom is that males are generally less socially skilled and adept than females, which means that autistic males are more likely to be accepted as socially inept. However, this can be an issue for autistic women who are expected to be socially competent. There may be concerns and potential conflict in the relationship regarding socializing with family and friends. For some autistic women, their partner may be their primary social relationship. However, their non-autistic partner probably anticipates more socializing than their autistic partner expects and can cope with.

Research by Crompton et al. (2020) explored the exhaustion and fatigue from socializing experienced by autistic women in a relationship. They complained that their non-autistic partner did not take autistic characteristics into account when organizing social events, such as the duration and number of people participating. The autistic women explained their difficulties reading facial expressions and intuitively knowing the unspoken social rules. The non-autistic partner can help explain social etiquette, how to make small talk and what is happening or going to happen in a social setting.

A characteristic we have noticed is autistic women disclosing too much information with friends, colleagues and strangers, seemingly unaware of social boundaries and expectations, which can be embarrassing, especially for the non-autistic partner. This requires the autistic woman's partner to be the social expert and have compassion for their difficulties in social situations.

An autistic woman may have learnt and achieved success in the art of flirting. However, she may use flirting in situations that would not be appropriate, such as when talking to the partner of a friend, or flirting with a stranger who may misinterpret this as a sign of seeking a sexual encounter.

The participants in the Crompton et al. study described increasing feelings of anxiety in advance of and during time with family and friends, as explained by one female autistic partner in the study: 'I get anxious because I have to behave well, to behave neurotypically, to do the right thing'. One research participant described subsequent exhaustion and emotional fatigue: 'Even if it is good, it is exhausting'. An autistic woman will probably have less social energy than her partner, and conflict can arise regarding when to leave a social gathering. We have found that autistic women, more than autistic men, can feel guilty for not being able to participate in social events or social conventions with their loved ones as much and as easily as their partner. The discrepancy between social capacity and social desire can lead to a feeling of loneliness, even when in a relationship.

We recognize that autism is associated with sensory sensitivity, but recent research has indicated that, in general, autistic women have greater sensory sensitivity than autistic men (Cardon et al., 2023). This can affect everyday life in terms of the acute discomfort or pain experienced with specific auditory sensory experiences, such as sudden or 'sharp' noises, for example a motorbike accelerating or someone shouting, visual sensitivity, especially light intensity, such as bright sunlight, olfactory sensitivity, for example perfumes and cleaning fluids, and tactile experiences such as labels and seams. The non-autistic partner may have difficulty appreciating the anticipatory anxiety of aversive sensory experiences of going to a shopping mall, a day on the beach and greeting a relative who wears strong perfumes. Tactile sensory sensitivity would also affect the experience of and response to gestures of reassurance and affection, such as gently touching an arm or hand and kissing. The withdrawal response is to the sensory experience rather than rejecting their partner's concern and compassion. Tactile sensitivity will also affect aspects of physical intimacy (see Chapter 15).

A central issue for relationship counselling is affection. Outdated societal expectations are that women should be affectionate and emotionally nurturing. The non-autistic partner may anticipate regular gestures and words of love and affection to occur for emotional repair and reassurance and, at times, to be simply spontaneous. An autistic woman may not read the signs that affection is anticipated or that affection would be an effective emotional repair. Subsequent conflict can be based on the expectation that, as a woman, she should intuitively know what her partner needs emotionally and how to respond.

There can be conflict in the relationship over the expression and reception of affection. Her non-autistic partner may assume affection and physical closeness would be effective and appreciated when she is distressed. However, she may feel overwhelmed by being touched, especially when distressed, and confused about how to respond to a hug or words of comfort and compassion. She may actively reject her partner's affection, who then feels personally rejected for being a caring and loving partner. An autistic woman will probably have solitary ways of emotionally de-stressing, repairing and recovering. The relationship counsellor will probably need to explain both partners' needs for expressions of affection but by different actions and intensity.

We have found that relationship counselling often includes exploring, giving and receiving compliments from both partner's perspectives. An autistic woman may find spontaneous compliments confusing, especially when compliments are not honest or a 'white lie'. They may also not recognize the importance and value of compliments within the relationship. This may give the non-autistic partner the impression that their autistic partner is emotionally cold and indifferent to their achievements. A cultural expectation is that women are expected to be almost effusive with their praise and compliments to their partner. The relationship counsellor may need to explain this characteristic of autism as a difficulty understanding the value of compliments in a relationship and providing advice on when and how to give a compliment.

Autism is associated with high levels of anxiety, and an autistic woman's partner will probably need to help her cope with situations such as a train being late, being in a crowd, an unexpected change and what may be considered trivial if not amusing by other people such as a missing apostrophe in a grocer's sign. Their partner will need to understand her thought processes and develop ways of soothing, distracting and emotionally regulating to a greater extent than anticipated in a non-autistic relationship.

REFERENCES

Cardon, G., Miranda McQuarrie, S., Calton, S., & Gabrielsen, T. P. (2023). Similar overall expression, but different profiles, of autistic traits, sensory processing, and mental health between young adult males and females. *Research in Autism Spectrum Disorders, 109*, 102263. https://doi.org/10.1016/j.rasd.2023.102263

Crompton, C. J., Hallett, S., Ropar, D., Flynn, E., & Fletcher-Watson, S. (2020). 'I never realised everybody felt as happy as I do when I am around autistic people': A thematic analysis of autistic adults' relationships with autistic and neurotypical friends and family. *Autism, 24*(6), 1438–1448. https://doi.org/10.1177/1362361320908976

Gibbs, V., Hudson, J., Hwang, Y. I., Arnold, S., Trollor, J., & Pellicano, E. (2021). Experiences of physical and sexual violence as reported by autistic adults without intellectual disability: Rate, gender patterns and clinical correlates. *Research in Autism Spectrum Disorders, 89*, 101866. https://doi.org/10.1016/j.rasd.2021.101866

Lai, M.-C., Lombardo, M. V., Ruigrok, A. N., Chakrabarti, B., Auyeung, B., Szatmari, P., Happé, F., & Baron-Cohen, S. (2017). Quantifying and exploring camouflaging in men and women with autism. *Autism, 21*(6), 690–702. https://doi.org/10.1177/1362361316671012

Pecora, L., Hancock, G., Hooley, M., Demmer, D., Mesibov, G., Attwood, T., & Stokes, M. A. (2020). Gender identity, sexual orientation and adverse sexual experiences in autistic females. *Molecular Autism, 11*. https://doi.org/10.1186/s13229-020-00363-0

Posserud, M.-B., Skretting Solberg, B., Engeland, A., Haavik, J., & Klungsøyr, K. (2021). Male to female ratios in autism spectrum disorders by age, intellectual disability and attention-deficit/hyperactivity disorder. *Acta Psychiatrica Scandinavica, 144*, 635–646. https://doi.org/10.1111/acps.13368

Sedgewick, F., Crane, L., Hill, V., & Pellicano, E. (2019). Friends and lovers: The relationships of autistic and neurotypical women. *Autism in Adulthood, 1*(2), 98–107. https://doi.org/10.1089/aut.2018.0028

CHAPTER 15

Intimacy, Sex and Sensory Sensitivity

Within the responses to our research, the sexual side of their relationship was not raised as something that was of concern by any of the autistic respondents. Only four non-autistic respondents revealed the sexual side of their relationship as something that was raised in their counselling sessions as problematic. This figure is very low, considering there were 184 respondents in this group. Two of these four stated that the counselling they received made matters worse. This is clearly shown in the quotes below:

> (NAFP) 'I was told to basically suck it up buttercup. Even with regards to my husband's sexually invasive behaviour. That was not helpful, especially while recovering from PTSD due to an unrelated matter'.

> (NAFP) 'After having my wifely role prescribed to me (stop your belly aching) and sent home with advice about sex, I was so nauseated by the sexual encounters that I became unable to have sex anymore'.

We do not know what the specific issue was that was raised by these respondents in the relationship counselling, but both these quotes strongly indicate that the advice that was received from the counsellors severely lacked the understanding of working with autistic neurodiverse couples. There has been very little research into the area of the sexual side of neurodiverse relationships and whether they should be regarded as any different from neurotypical relationships.

A study that investigated relationship satisfaction in autistic and non-autistic individuals in long-term relationships found that a higher relationship and sexual satisfaction was reported in the autistic group compared to the non-autistic group (Yew et al., 2023). This is backed up by the findings in our survey, as difficulties surrounding the sexual side of the relationship were only raised by the non-autistic partner.

Another reason for the non-autistic partner to score low on sexual desire and satisfaction can be due to the lack of emotional support and connection they receive from their partner. This was expressed by some non-autistic partners as the barrier to their achieving sexual satisfaction. Once again, this is described in the quotes below:

> (NAFP) 'Three-minute encounters never worked for me. My spouse could never understand that maintaining an emotional relationship required some time'.

> (NAFP) 'I adjusted to the way things are, but grieve a lack of emotional intimacy'.

Relationship counselling will need to address this imbalance between emotional intimacy and sexual connection. Finding ways to balance emotional and physical intimacy can be a challenge. The counsellor will need to explain this in a way that the autistic partner can relate to.

Finding an appropriate analogy for this can be useful. We have found that using the analogy of sharing a meal can be easily related to and applied to sharing sexual encounters. The description can be offered by comparing the difference between eating a quick snack or takeaway and taking the time to prepare and share a three-course meal.

Sometimes, a quick takeaway suffices, especially if time is limited or the purpose is simply to satisfy a physical need. There are also times when it is important to take the time together to share a three-course meal and spend quality time preparing the food, setting the scene and savouring every mouthful together. The result of this will be that both partners will feel connected, contented and nurtured, not unlike spending time over sharing sex together.

Using this analogy can be useful as it brings home the relevance that the sexual act begins long before penetrative sex or before reaching an orgasm, and neither should it immediately end after this has been achieved. This can mean planning, preparing, cooking and setting the scene, representing the quality time spent together sharing and valuing each other's contribution. The starter is the foreplay, which is crucial to tantalizing and teasing the appetite for what is to come. The main meal is the sharing of the ultimate sexual connection, experiencing the peaks of excitement before reaching an orgasm. The dessert is the winding down, the time to compliment and show appreciation to each other for the trust and privilege of sharing one's body with another.

Taking the time to share together and enjoy all aspects of the sexual union is vital if both an emotional and satisfying physical connection is going to be achieved by the couple. Relationship counselling will need to explore what each meal course means to each partner, as both may express very different needs and expectations. Finding a way to satisfy both may take time, understanding and patience. Once achieved, though, this can greatly improve the couple's relationship. However, whether it can be achieved will depend on several factors, and one very important factor for relationship counselling to consider is whether the autistic partner is struggling with issues caused by sensory sensitivity.

Sensory sensitivity and how it affects each autistic individual can play a major role in determining sexual satisfaction in a relationship (Aston, 2012a). This area will need to be explored in detail by the counsellor before any exercises involving physical connection are given to the couple.

A study which explored the sexual experience of 24 autistic adults found that every one of their participants struggled with sensory regulation issues, which often left them feeling emotionally upset or in physical pain (Barnett & Maticka-Tyndale, 2015). The implications behind these findings validate the importance of exploring this area with the autistic partner.

In addition to difficulties managing sensory dysregulation, the study also found that there was sometimes a delay in conveying this information to the non-autistic sexual partner, and this is described adequately in the quote below from a 39-year-old autistic heterosexual woman:

> Sometimes I will realise that I've been gritting my teeth and enduring something unpleasant for five minutes without noticing it, before I get my act together to push someone's hand away or ask for a different kind of touch. (Barnett & Maticka-Tyndale, 2015, p. 174)

This could cause confusion for the non-autistic partner, especially when they discover that rather than the pleasure they thought they were giving their partner, they were causing them pain. This will be particularly the case if there is no understanding of autism and sensory sensitivity. Time will need to be taken to explain this, and reassurance will need to be given to the non-autistic partner that they are not being blamed. Reminding them that they were unaware that their attempts to stimulate their partner were, in fact, being experienced as painful or unpleasant.

Sensory sensitivity can take many forms and have various levels of severity, from mildly uncomfortable to excruciatingly painful. Using a table of numbers 0 to 10 can be useful here to help the autistic partner label how painful or uncomfortable an experience is for them. Ten would be the most painful, and zero would be no pain at all. An alternative to this could be to use a series of emoji faces that go from a calm face to a painful face. Once again, relationship counselling will need to explore with the couple what works best for them.

Making use of a body chart (Aston, 2021, pp. 136–140) can be invaluable in helping the autistic partner to illustrate the sensitive areas of their body and, in addition, the type of their preferred touch. This can come as a great relief for both partners and remove the guesswork from their sexual encounters.

For some autistic individuals, the difficulties they experience may not always be limited to touch; they may be due to taste, smell and visual senses. All senses have a role in sexual encounters. All will need to be explored within the relationship counselling.

A non-autistic husband was very confused as to why his wife would not let him kiss her on her mouth. He was able to kiss her on her body but stated she showed absolute repulsion if he attempted to kiss her on her lips. After much reassurance that he would not be offended by her reply, she shared that she found the smell of his breath nauseating, even though his breath odour was quite normal. Her heightened sense of smell found his breath, and anyone else's breath, very unpleasant, which had been the case since she was a child.

Once this was understood, the expectation that he could kiss his wife on her lips was removed. He no longer felt rejected because he understood it was not personal. Very often, once the reason behind a behaviour is understood, it no longer presents as confusing or threatening. Feelings of rejection or being offended can be left behind, and the focus can be placed on what is working and going well.

Another area for relationship counselling to explore is the environment in which the couple have sex. Checking out sensitivity to the lights in the room, the smells of perfume, aftershave or scented candles, and the feel of fabrics, such as nightwear or bed sheets, are just some of the areas to investigate. These important factors are sometimes regarded as trivial, but to an autistic individual, they are crucial, as they can be a cause of distraction, irritation and an inability to enjoy the sex they are sharing.

Turner et al. (2019) found that autistic men scored higher on sexual excitement and arousal scores compared to the scores found within the general population when applying the dual control model of sexual response (Bancroft et al., 2009; Janssen & Bancroft, 2023). Some autistic adults described how, due to hypersensitivity, they could find that even non-sexual touch was strongly arousing. However, it was also found that maintaining this level of excitement during sex could be problematic, and their arousal level could fade as quickly as it came. This was considered to be due to the decrease in stimulation during sex, thus making it difficult to maintain an erection (Turner et al., 2019). As it is not always possible to maintain continuous and stronger pressure during sex, issues around erectile functioning were found among the autistic participants.

In our experience, we have found that for some autistic partners there can be a preference for masturbation rather than sharing penetrative sex with their partner. Some have described that achieving sexual gratification via masturbation is much easier and less stressful than trying to initiate sex with their partner. Masturbation can sometimes be viewed quite objectively, as simply being a means to an end that does not require getting the timing right, reading their partner's needs and having to provide any emotional input.

Sarah Hendrix includes the following quotes in her book:

> For many years, my husband (AS) preferred to masturbate 5+ times a week whilst rejecting my advances. After many tears and some counselling, he stopped masturbating but seems to have chosen celibacy instead. (NT female). (Hendrix, 2008, p. 72)

> I masturbate about three times a week. I haven't had sex with my wife in three years (since our wedding night). (AS male). (Hendrix, 2008, p. 73)

In contrast, autistic women were more likely to be hyposensitive when it came to becoming sexually aroused, and some reported needing very intense stimulation to be able to reach a clitoral orgasm.

Scores for sexual excitement were reported lower for women than men; this could, however, be due to being hypersensitive in the vaginal area, causing penetration to be painful. For some autistic women, hypersensitivity can produce vaginal muscle spasms. This painful condition is known as vaginismus and can be difficult to treat if this is the cause.

If this is an area for concern raised in relationship counselling, then, unless the counsellor is also a psychosexual therapist, it might prove beneficial to the client to be referred to a therapist who is qualified in this domain and also very knowledgeable about working with autistic women.

In addition, painful intercourse may also be due to tension and anxiety. It should be noted that a very high percentage of autistic women fall victim to sexual abuse (Cazalis et al., 2022), and this could explain the reason behind the higher sexual inhibition scores by the women in the study (Turner et al., 2019). If the issue of past sexual abuse is raised in relationship counselling, then an individual session (if preferred) should be offered to the client. This applies to either partner. However, if the partner is autistic, the counsellor may need to take time to sensitively explore this, as it may not have been recognized that the behaviour towards them was abusive and they are not responsible.

Issues regarding the use of pornography and sexual deviance were not raised within our survey by the couples who responded. However, we are both aware from our work with couples that this is an area that can present as a problem between neurodiverse couples and one we have discussed in our previous publications (Aston, 2012b; Attwood, 2006).

Seeking out pornography, sexual deviance and paraphilic behaviour exists within all populations worldwide regardless of race, gender, sexuality or gender identification. Research has, though, indicated that some behaviours are more likely to occur among autistic adults when compared to non-autistic adults (Schöttle et al., 2017; Turner et al., 2019). The behaviours which were found to be significantly higher were those of the voyeuristic, fetishist and masochistic types (Fernandes et al., 2016; Schottle et al., 2017). Research into this area is still greatly lacking; however, drawing on the research available, it appears that the reasons and causes behind these behaviours are likely to be different compared to the non-autistic population (Gray et al., 2021; Schottle et al., 2017; Turner et al., 2019). These findings concur with what we have also found in our work with couples (Aston, 2012a, 2012b; Attwood, 2006).

These differences are very important for relationship counsellors and psychosexual therapists to be aware of when working with autistic individuals and couples. It is imperative that the counsellor/therapist is able to share their understanding with the couple they are working with, as only then will the couple be able to manage the issues that are causing them concern and impacting their relationship. This particularly applies to the use of pornography.

It has been argued that there is little to separate voyeurism from watching pornographic videos, as both often occur in secret, especially when watching pornography is a solitary pursuit and one which is not supported by their partner. We have both worked with couples when the watching of pornography by the autistic male partner has been discovered by the non-autistic partner and resulted in very negative consequences for the relationship and been the primary reason for couple counselling to be sought.

The discovery that a partner has been watching pornography can, for some, feel as much like a betrayal as an affair. Most devastating is the loss of trust, especially if promises to stop are made and then broken. In the majority of the couples we have worked with, it has been the male autistic partner who has been discovered watching pornography, and the reaction to the discovery has been varied. The most common reaction has been surprise that their partner is so upset (Aston, 2012b), and rather than show remorse, they have reacted with a counterargument that they have not been unfaithful. Some have shown even more surprise that their partner did not share their curiosity and wish to share in what, for many, had become a special interest.

Watching pornography has also been used by autistic partners for what they consider to be educational reasons and a desire to enhance their sexual performance. Their intimate partner may be the only partner they have shared sex with, and therefore have very limited experience and understanding of sexual intimacy. The danger with using internet pornography is that it can lead to the observer being misinformed and can result in inappropriate sexual behaviours and expectations.

Relationship counselling will need to spend time exploring the reasons why pornography was being used. The counsellor should try to discover whether it was to gain sexual experience and, if so, what was their understanding of what they observed.

Exploration as to whether pornography has developed into a special interest is also relevant for relationship counselling to explore, and if so, what aspect of pornography is the interest linked to? It may be discovered that there is an interest in breast size, specifically areola shape and

RELATIONSHIP COUNSELLING WITH AUTISTIC NEURODIVERSE COUPLES

size. Sometimes, it can just be accumulating vast collections of photos of specific body parts and not always linked to sexual excitement.

Watching pornography can also be used to accompany masturbation, and this may be the partner's preferred way to achieve sexual stimulation and release. This can be particularly devastating to their partner, who may have been sacrificing a sexual life for years with no understanding of why. The reasons for this are hypersensitivity, as we discussed earlier in this chapter. It is being increasingly discovered in research that hyper- and hyposensitivity might be responsible for many other sexual behaviours and, in some cases, a complete withdrawal from any sexual activity (Gray et al., 2021), and if this appears to be of concern to a couple then relationship counselling will need to explore this with them. The primary focus in relationship counselling is to ensure that neither partner is being coerced or having to endure a behaviour which they find painful or uncomfortable. If this is the case, we recommend offering an individual session with the client.

Sex is a form of communication, and greater amounts of sexual communication increase sexual satisfaction in both partners and have been associated with increased orgasm frequency in women (Jones et al., 2018). Unfortunately, as we have already discussed, difficulties in communication and reading the non-verbal signals in communication can be very problematic for the autistic partner. Sex signals and indicators are rarely spoken and rely on non-verbal communication. This can prove very difficult for the autistic partner, who may misread their partner's intentions. This can include believing that sex is being offered by their partner when they only want a hug, or missing the signals altogether and ignoring signs that their partner would like to have sex with them. Both these scenarios can cause misunderstandings, confusion and some very hurt feelings in the relationship.

Relationship counselling will need to work with the couple on finding other ways besides non-verbal guides to indicate whether the non-autistic partner is in the mood for sex. There are various ways this can be achieved, such as using colours, numbers and wearing specific nightwear. The counsellor will need to discover what would work reliably and safely for the couple. It is worth making the rule with the couple that a hug does not mean wanting sex, as signs of affection can be easily misinterpreted by the autistic partner as an indication of sexual desire.

In our work with couples, we found that for many, the sexual side of the relationship was quite positive and satisfying, especially if the couple shared a similar appetite for sex, regardless of whether that meant sex was frequent or infrequent. As long as the couple's needs were compatible, then the sexual side of the relationship was rarely the issue that was brought to counselling.

We did, though, find that for some autistic partners, sex became their special interest, and some spent much time reading and learning about how to make it as good as possible, and some achieved this very well. However, once the autistic partner feels that the sexual act has reached its peak of perfection, the non-autistic partner might find there is a strong resistance to making any changes. Any suggestion they make to try something different could be interpreted by their partner as a form of criticism. One gentleman became very upset and confused when his partner suggested they try something new. He felt betrayed by his partner and stated that they had told him in the past that it had been the best sex they had ever experienced. He could not understand why they would say such a thing and then suggest they do something different. Once again, the analogy of a meal might help the counsellor to explain this to the autistic partner, in that although a meal might perfect in every way, if eaten every day, it may become monotonous. It is more stimulating to have a variety of meals to enjoy and share together.

Studies into relationships have found that couples who share a sense of humour are the most likely to succeed in having a long-term and happy relationship (Łukasz et al., 2022). This applies equally to neurodiverse couples, and if relationship counselling can draw out this side of the couple and find ways for the couple to bring some fun and enjoyment into their sex life, then this will be of benefit to both partners.

REFERENCES

Aston, M. (2012a). Asperger syndrome in the bedroom. *Sexual and Relationship Therapy, 27*(1), 73–72.

Aston, M. (2012b). *What men with Asperger syndrome want to know about women, dating and relationships*. Jessica Kingsley Publishers.

Aston, M. (2021). *The autism couple's workbook* (2nd ed.). Jessica Kingsley Publishers.

Attwood, T. (2006). *The complete guide to Asperger syndrome*. Jessica Kingsley Publishers.

Bancroft, J., Graham, C. A., Janssen, E., & Sanders, S. A. (2009). The dual control model: Current status and future directions. *Journal of Sex Research, 46*(2–3), 121–142. https://doi.org/10.1080/00224490902747222

Barnett, J. P., & Maticka-Tyndale, E. (2015). Qualitative exploration of sexual experiences among adults on the autism spectrum: Implications for sex education. *Perspectives on Sexual and Reproductive Health, 47*(4), 171–179. https://doi.org/10.1363/47e5715

Cazalis, F., Reyes, E., Leduc, S., & Gourion, D. (2022). Evidence that nine autistic women out of ten have been victims of sexual violence. *Frontiers in Behavioral Neuroscience, 16,* 852203. https://doi.org/10.3389/fnbeh.2022.852203

Fernandes, L. C., Gillberg, C. I., Cederlund, M., Hagberg, B., Gillberg, C., & Billstedt, E. (2016). Aspects of sexuality in adolescents and adults diagnosed with autism spectrum disorders in childhood. *Journal of Autism and Developmental Disorders, 46,* 3155–3165. https://doi. org/10.1007/s10803-016-2855-9

Gray, S., Kirby, A. V., & Holmes, L. G. (2021). Autistic narratives of sensory features and relationships. *Autism in Adulthood, 3*(3). https://doi.org/10.1089/aut.2020.004

Hendrix, S. (2008). *Love, sex & long-term relationships.* Jessica Kingsley Publishers.

Janssen, E., & Bancroft, J. (2023). The dual control model of sexual response: A scoping review, 2009–2022. *Journal of Sex Research, 60*(7), 948–968. https://doi.org/10.1080/0 0224499.2023.2219247

Jones, A. C., Robinson, W. D., & Seedall, R. B. (2018). The role of sexual communication in couples' sexual outcomes: A dyadic path analysis. *Journal of Marital and Family Therapy, 44*(4), 606–623. https://doi.org/10.1111/jmft.12282

Łukasz, J., Kubicius, D., & Jonason, P. K. (2022). 'Do they fit together like the Joker and Harley Quinn?': Joking, laughing, humor styles, and dyadic adjustment among people in long-term romantic relationships. *Personality and Individual Differences, 199,* 111859. https:// doi.org/10.1016/j.paid.2022.111859

Schöttle, D., Briken, P., Tüscher, O., & Turner, D. (2017). Sexuality in autism: Hypersexual and paraphilic behavior in women and men with high-functioning autism spectrum disorder. *Dialogues in Clinical Neuroscience, 19*(4), 381–393. https://doi.org/10.31887/ DCNS.2017.19.4/

Turner, D., Briken, P., & Schöttle, D. (2019). Sexual dysfunctions and their association with the dual control model of sexual response in men and women with high-functioning autism. *Journal of Clinical Medicine, 8*(4), 425. https://doi.org/10.3390/jcm8040425

Yew, R. Y., Hooley, M., & Stokes, M. (2023). Factors of relationship satisfaction for autistic and non-autistic partners in long-term relationships. *Autism, 27*(8). https://doi. org/10.1177/13623613231160244

CHAPTER 16

Autism Plus

Autism often co-occurs with signs of other neurodevelopmental, psychiatric and medical conditions. These include attention deficit hyperactivity disorder (ADHD), mood disorders, especially anxiety disorders and depression, trauma, eating and personality disorders, substance abuse and specific medical conditions.

NEURODEVELOPMENTAL DISORDERS

The most common co-occurring neurodivergence with autism is ADHD. A recent meta-analysis indicates that 40–70% of autistic children and adults also have clinical signs of ADHD (Rong et al., 2021). The signs include difficulties regulating attention, being impulsive, having initial enthusiasm for an activity but lacking motivation to complete it, difficulties with organizational, planning and time management abilities, being distractable, a tendency to lose things, fidgeting and talking incessantly. There can also be a tendency to make careless mistakes and be notorious for interrupting.

All these characteristics will impact the relationship and create considerable stress, agitation and potential conflict for both partners. Psychologists describe this pattern of characteristics as impaired executive function, and the non-ADHD partner will often reluctantly become an executive secretary at home and exasperated by the additional responsibility and lack of significant progress in encouraging their autistic partner to improve their executive functioning abilities.

When autism and ADHD co-occur, relationship counselling will need to explore how problems with executive functioning affect the relationship and how both partners can adjust to and accommodate the characteristics of ADHD. Many books are now available on understanding and living with ADHD. Relationship counselling should encourage both partners to develop their understanding of how it will impact their relationship. Psychologists and psychiatrists are increasingly identifying adults who have ADHD and providing appropriate support, therapy and, if necessary, medication.

Other co-occurring neurodivergent conditions associated with autism include dyslexia, dyscalculia and dyspraxia. These may have significantly impacted the autistic partner's school and adult years. If written material is used during counselling, it is important to enquire if the client has any reading difficulties or dyspraxia, which may affect handwriting when completing some counselling activities, with a preference for typing rather than writing.

Around 10% of autistic adults will have a tic disorder, from occasional motor and vocal tics to Tourette's syndrome (Kalyva et al., 2016). Common tics are blinking, coughing, throat clearing, sniffing and facial movements. Tics may commence in childhood and decrease during adolescence but may continue in the adult years. There is no effective medication, but behavioural therapies can temporarily suppress the urge to engage in tic behaviour. The tics are perceived as benign in terms of psychopathology but can be irritating for the non-autistic partner, who may need encouragement to be tolerant and not get distracted by the tics.

PSYCHIATRIC DISORDERS

A recent study confirmed that nearly 80% of autistic adults will meet the criteria for a psychiatric disorder at least once in their lives (Lever & Geurts, 2016). The most common psychiatric disorders are anxiety disorders and depression, trauma, eating and personality disorders and substance abuse.

Anxiety

Almost 40% of autistic adults experience a moderate to severe anxiety disorder during their lifetime (Murray et al., 2019), and 86% have daily problems with anxiety (Evans et al., 2014). All expressions of anxiety are associated with autism, including generalized anxiety disorder with excessive worry about upcoming events, obsessive-compulsive disorder (OCD) with compulsive behaviour and thoughts, social anxiety, which includes worry about social performance, evaluation and acceptance, as well as phobias, which can be caused by anxiety due to anticipated aversive sensory experiences such as loud noises, bright lights and tactile experiences.

A relationship counsellor will likely have previously experienced anxious clients, but autistic adults may have greater and more specific anxiety associated with aspects of counselling. Their generalized anxiety can build prior to the counselling session such that they are extremely anxious when they walk into the counselling room. It would be appropriate first to check the person's anxiety level and consider ways to reduce it, such as breathing activities, before starting the counselling. The level of generalized anxiety during the session can make an autistic client more 'rigid' and less 'flexible' in their thinking and ability to perceive alternative perspectives and options. OCD may be expressed as a ritual action that must be completed to reduce anxiety, such as touching a wooden surface, stroking an item of clothing or a compulsion to complete an activity in the session. The relationship counsellor will become aware of the signs of OCD and either accept them as a means of reducing anxiety or suggest alternative means of anxiety reduction. Social anxiety can be anxiety due to not having had previous experience with counselling and being unsure of their role, as well as expectations and conventions in a new social situation. They may feel uncomfortable when the centre of attention, and autism is associated with situational mutism; that is, the person is so anxious they are physically unable to talk. There may be a phobia of items in the counselling room due to sensory sensitivity, such as hearing the sound of the fan in a computer, bright sunlight on their face or the texture of the furniture fabric. Environmental modifications may be needed to reduce anxiety levels.

Depression

Over 45% of autistic adults experience moderate to severe depression during their lifetime (Murray et al., 2019), and 76% have daily problems with depressed mood (Evans et al., 2014). An analysis of coroners' inquest records and interviews with next of kin of those who committed suicide found that 41% of those who died were autistic or had elevated autistic traits (Cassidy et al., 2022).

An autistic life is not an easy life. There are many reasons for the association between autism and depression, including genetics, chronic exhaustion from trying to cope with social and sensory experiences, being misunderstood and criticized, exhaustion from high levels of anxiety, feeling lonely even in a relationship and disappointing their partner, believing that past bad experiences will continue forever, coping with too many expectations at home and work and not having enough strategies or experiences to feel happy again.

Depression will affect energy and commitment levels within relationship counselling sessions and when applying new relationship abilities with their partner. Both the relationship counsellor and the non-autistic partner could be concerned about the prevalence of pessimism, negativity and suicidal thoughts. When there are mild signs of depression, there are self-help programmes specifically designed for autistic adults (Attwood & Garnett, 2016), and greater signs would indicate that the autistic partner needs to seek psychiatric help.

Trauma

Around 30% to 45% of autistic adults have probable post-traumatic stress disorder (PTSD) compared to 4% of the non-autistic population (Haruvi-Lamdan et al., 2018; Rumball et al., 2021). An autistic partner may have had exposure to multiple traumatic events, including physical, emotional and sexual abuse and other negative life events. Often, the most distressing event is social, from bullying and teasing to physical and sexual assault. These two studies of autism and PTSD found no gender differences in the frequency and trauma types and confirmed that PTSD can exacerbate certain autistic traits, including social withdrawal, emotion regulation difficulties and sleep problems. The first disclosure of having experienced trauma and abuse may occur during relationship counselling, and the counsellor will need to take appropriate action. There is research evidence that eye movement desensitization and reprocessing can be successful in reducing the signs of PTSD in autistic adults (Lobregt-van Buuren et al., 2019).

Eating and Personality Disorders

We know that over 30% of adolescents with an eating disorder are autistic (Brede et al., 2020) and that an eating disorder may have been a significant psychiatric experience for an autistic partner, with current or residual issues in the adult years. The presence of an eating disorder, past or present, will impact the relationship. If it becomes apparent in the relationship counselling that the eating disorder is the dominant cause of the disharmony between the couple, it should be considered by the relationship counsellor in supervision as to whether the client in question should be referred to a specialist in this area.

The profile of adaptations to being autistic can lead to a current or previous diagnosis of a personality disorder. This can include borderline personality disorder (BPD) with a fear of abandonment, intense personal relationships and extremes of idealization and devaluation, suicidal behaviour, anger management issues and chronic feelings of emptiness. This is a more likely to be diagnosed in an autistic female than a male (May et al., 2021). BPD appears to be the diagnosis frequently given to women before the correct diagnosis of autism is discovered. This could be due to a lack of awareness of how autism affects autistic women and the fact that until recently the diagnostic criteria available to clinicians were specifically designed for autistic men. Misdiagnosis could also be due to the ability of autistic women to mask their autism. It is important for the counsellor to be open to the fact that they may be working with a client who has been misdiagnosed. If the client is also of the same opinion, it may be appropriate to recommend that they check this with their GP or seek a referral to a clinical psychologist or psychiatrist. The fear of abandonment and extremes of adulation and denigration may be factors identified during relationship counselling. There are a range of treatment options for BPD, including dialectical behaviour therapy.

The personality of autistic adults could resemble paranoid personality disorder due to the experience of rejection and bullying by peers in childhood. The distrust and suspiciousness may be well founded on past experience and be an aspect of the relationship. Schizoid personality disorder can describe someone who chooses to be detached from social relationships and has a restricted range of emotions in interpersonal settings. This can also be a description of some autistic adults. A lack of friendships and social achievements in childhood, as well as reduced cognitive and behavioural empathy and a tendency to escape into a fantasy world, could lead to the consideration of narcissistic personality disorder. This may be a compensation mechanism with the creation of a grandiose sense of self-importance, fantasies regarding success, power and brilliance, and requiring excessive admiration with a sense of entitlement and arrogance. A non-autistic partner may describe their autistic partner as sometimes being a narcissist.

Although it is possible to be both autistic and narcissistic, this is not always the case. Confusion can come from the sometimes-self-absorbed nature of the autistic partner, and it can feel that their priorities are very self-centred and do not accommodate their partner's feelings or needs.

This will be to an even greater degree if the autistic partner is in denial of being neurodiverse, and, in order to maintain this, will behave in a way that can outwardly appear as sanctimonious.

Substance Abuse

Up to 36% of autistic adults have problems with substance abuse (But-wicka et al., 2017; Ressel et al., 2020), which may be a way of engaging or escaping reality. The starting point is often alcohol and marijuana, which can act as a social 'lubricant' and reduce social anxiety, thereby facilitating an autistic adolescent's or adult's social engagement. The risk is that the person becomes dependent on alcohol and marijuana to lower anxiety generally and especially in social situations. Autistic adults can have difficulty relaxing and may not consider or be responsive to interpersonal means of relaxation. Both substances are effective relaxants and can enhance positive feelings. There is also an association between autism and heavy episodic drinking (Brosnan & Adams, 2020). Legal and illegal mood-altering substances can also be used to disengage socially, creating emotional detachment from current circumstances and being 'anaesthetized' from past trauma. The substances slow down racing and anxious thoughts and reduce stress.

Substance abuse will affect the relationship as recognized by an experienced relationship counsellor. If the substance abuse is ongoing, then the addicted partner would need to be referred to a specialist group or professional working in this area. Substance abuse will impair emotion regulation and decision making and can be a factor in domestic violence. Substance abuse could also potentially lead to entry into the criminal justice system. Treatment, especially residential rehabilitation for substance abuse in an autistic adult, will need to be adjusted to accommodate the experiences and ability profile associated with autism.

MEDICAL CONDITIONS

There are a range of medical conditions associated with autism. The most common is insomnia, which is caused by difficulties falling asleep, staying asleep, and the quality of sleep for autistic individuals of all ages (Bishop-Fitzpatrick & Rubenstein, 2019; Stewart et al., 2022). Research indicates that sleep problems may not have been assessed by a healthcare professional (Halstead et al., 2021). Sleep issues will have an impact on the relationship and may need to be addressed by a physician.

There is a marginally greater risk of autoimmune conditions such as psoriasis and asthma, gastrointestinal conditions and stress-related illnesses (Bougeard et al., 2021) and Ehlers-Danlos syndrome (Kindgren et al., 2021). There can also be a high pain threshold and a high frequency of migraines. There is also a marginally greater prevalence of dementia (Vivanti et al., 2021) and Parkinson's disease (Geurts et al., 2022), and around 8% of intellectually able autistic adults have epilepsy (Liu et al., 2022).

In recent years, there has been an increased prevalence of autistic adolescents and adults seeking and achieving gender transformation. Recent research indicates that between 5 and 26% of those attending a gender clinic for adults are autistic (Cheung et al., 2018). The autistic partner may be considering changing gender or have changed gender. The relationship counsellor will need to consider gender dysphoria as a factor in such relationships in terms of gender experiences and expectations for both partners and adjust counselling accordingly.

Thus, for clients who have a formal diagnosis of autism or have significant autistic characteristics, the relationship counsellor will need to be aware of the additional neurodevelopmental, psychiatric and medical conditions associated with autism and their impact on the relationship.

REFERENCES

Attwood, T., & Garnett, M. (2016). *Exploring depression and beating the blues*. Jessica Kingsley Publishers.

Bishop-Fitzpatrick, L., & Rubenstein, E. (2019). The physical and mental health of middle-aged and older adults on the autism spectrum and the impact of intellectual disability. *Research in Autism Spectrum Disorders, 63*, 34–41. https://doi.org/10.1016/j.rasd.2019.01.001

Bougeard, C., Picarel-Blanchot, F., Schmid, R., Campbell, R., & Buitelaar, J. (2021). Prevalence of autism spectrum disorder and co-morbidities in children and adolescents: A systematic review of the literature. *Frontiers in Psychiatry, 9*, Article 751. https://doi.org/10.3389/fpsyt.2021.744709

Brede, J., Babb, C., Jones, C., Elliott, M., Zanker, C., Tchanturia, K., Serpell, L., Fox, J., & Mandy, W. (2020). 'For me, the anorexia is just a symptom, and the cause is the autism': Investigating restrictive eating disorders in autistic women. *Journal of Autism and Developmental Disorders, 50*, 4280–4296. https://doi.org/10.1007/s10803-020-04479-3

Brosnan, M., & Adams, S. (2020). The expectancies and motivations for heavy episodic drinking of alcohol in autistic adults. *Autism in Adulthood, 2*, 317–324. https://doi.org/10.1089/aut.2020.0008

Butwicka, A., Långström, N., Larsson, H., Lundström, S., Serlachius, E., Almqvist, C., Frisén, L., & Lichtenstein, P. (2017). Increased risk for substance use-related problems in autism spectrum disorders: A population-based cohort study. *Journal of Autism and Developmental Disorders, 47*, 80–89. https://doi.org/10.1007/s10803-016-2914-2

Cassidy, S., Au-Yeung, S., Robertson, A., Cogger-Ward, H., Richards, G., Allison, C., Bradley, L., Kenny, R., O'Connor, R., Mosse, D., Rodgers, J., & Baron-Cohen, S. (2022). Autism and autistic traits in those who died by suicide. *The British Journal of Psychiatry, 221,* 683–691. https://doi.org/10.1192/bjp.2022.21

Cheung, A., Ooi, O., Leemaqz, S., Cundill, P., Silberstein, N., Bretherton, I., Thrower, E., Locke, P., Grossmann, M., & Zajac, J. D. (2018). Sociodemographic and clinical characteristics of transgender adults in Australia. *Transgender Health, 3,* 229–238.

Evans, C., Lesko, A., & Attwood, A. (Eds.). (2014). *Been there. Done that. Try this!* Jessica Kingsley Publishers.

Geurts, H. M., McQuaid, G. A., Begeer, S., & Wallace, G. L. (2022). Self-reported parkinsonism features in older autistic adults: A descriptive study. *Autism, 26*(1), 217–229. https://doi.org/10.1177/13623613211020183

Halstead, E., Sullivan, E., Zambelli, Z., Ellis, J. G., & Dimitriou, D. (2021). The treatment of sleep problems in autistic adults in the United Kingdom. *Autism, 25*(8), 2412–2417. https://doi.org/10.1177/13623613211007226

Haruvi-Lamdan, N., Horesh, D., & Golan, O. (2018). PTSD and autism spectrum disorder: Co-morbidity, gaps in research, and potential shared mechanisms. *Psychological Trauma: Theory, Research, Practice, and Policy, 10*(3), 290–299. https://doi.org/10.1037/tra0000298

Kalyva, E., Kyriazi, M., Vargiami, E., & Zafeiriou, D. I. (2016). A review of co-occurrence of autism spectrum disorder and Tourette syndrome. *Research in Autism Spectrum Disorders, 24,* 39–51. https://doi.org/10.1016/j.rasd.2016.01.007

Kindgren, E., Quiñones Perez, A., & Knez, R. (2021). Prevalence of ADHD and autism spectrum disorder in children with hypermobility spectrum disorders or hypermobile Ehlers-Danlos syndrome: A retrospective study. *Neuropsychiatric Disease and Treatment, 10,* 379–388. https://doi.org/10.2147/NDT.S290494

Lever, A. G., & Geurts, H. M. (2016). Psychiatric co-occurring symptoms and disorders in young, middle-aged, and older adults with autism spectrum disorder. *Journal of Autism and Developmental Disorders, 46,* 1916–1930. https://doi.org/10.1007/s10803-016-2722-8

Liu, X., Sun, X., Sun, C., Zou, M., Chen, Y., Huang, J., Wu, L., & Chen, W. X. (2022). Prevalence of epilepsy in autism spectrum disorders: A systematic review and meta-analysis. *Autism, 26*(1), 33–50.

Lobregt-van Buuren, E., Sizoo, B., Mevissen, L., & de Jongh, A. (2019). Eye movement desensitization and reprocessing (EMDR) therapy as a feasible and potential effective treatment for adults with autism spectrum disorder (ASD) and a history of adverse events. *Journal of Autism and Developmental Disorders, 49,* 151–164. https://doi.org/10.1007/s10803-018-3687-6

May, T., Pilkington, P. D., Younan, R., & Williams, K. (2021). Overlap of autism spectrum disorder and borderline personality disorder: A systematic review and meta-analysis. *Autism Research, 14,* 2688–2710. https://doi.org/10.1002/aur.2619

Murray, C., Kovshoff, H., Brown, A., Abbott, P., & Hadwin, J. A. (2019). Exploring the anxiety and depression profile in individuals diagnosed with an autism spectrum disorder in adulthood. *Research in Autism Spectrum Disorders, 58,* 1–8. https://doi.org/10.1016/j.rasd.2018.11.002

Ressel, M., Thompson, B., Poulin, M.-H., Normand, C. L., Fisher, M. H., Couture, G., & Iarocci, G. (2020). Systematic review of risk and protective factors associated with substance use and abuse in individuals with autism spectrum disorders. *Autism, 24*(4), 899–918. https://doi.org/10.1177/1362361320910963

Rong, Y., Yang, C.-J., Jin, Y., & Wang, Y. (2021). Prevalence of attention-deficit/hyperactivity disorder in individuals with autism spectrum disorder: A meta-analysis. *Research in Autism Spectrum Disorders, 83,* 1750–9467. https://doi.org/10.1016/j.rasd.2021.101759

Rumball, F., Brook, L., Happé, F., & Karl, A. (2021). Heightened risk of posttraumatic stress disorder in adults with autism spectrum disorder: The role of cumulative trauma and memory deficits. *Research in Developmental Disabilities, 110,* 103848. https://doi.org/10.1016/j.ridd.2020.103848

Stewart, T. M., Martin, K., Fazi, M., Oldridge, J., Piper, A., & Rhodes, S. M. (2022). A systematic review of the rates of depression in autistic children and adolescents without intellectual disability. *Psychology and Psychotherapy, 95*(1), 313–344. https://doi.org/10.1111/papt.12366

Vivanti, G., Sha Tao, K., Lyall, K., Robins, D. L., & Shea, L. L. (2021). The prevalence and incidence of early-onset dementia among adults with autism spectrum disorder. *Autism Research, 14*, 2189–2199. https://doi.org/10.1002/aur.2590

Working with Autistic Neurodiverse Relationships

CHAPTER 17

What to Consider Before Working with Neurodiverse Couples

CONSIDER PROFESSIONAL COMPETENCE

At this present time, there is no specific qualification requirement for a counsellor to work with autistic individuals, couples or families. In other words, a counsellor with no prior training, knowledge or personal experience of autism could effectively advertise as working in this area and see autistic clients for counselling. Maxine recalls once being told by an experienced counselling supervisor that it was totally irrelevant whether a client was autistic, and this should not be of concern to the counsellor or the counselling!

The results from this survey highlighted just how important it is for a counsellor to be knowledgeable, and the reports we received showed links between a counsellor's experience and training and whether the counselling was beneficial and the outcome successful. Before deciding to work with autistic individuals, a counsellor has an ethical requirement to consider whether they can offer their clients genuine understanding and supply the appropriate support the couple needs to achieve positive change and rectifications in their relationship.

For some counsellors, their experience of autism has been developed on a personal level. This could be due to having a parent, partner or child who is autistic. The personal lived experience of autism is very valuable. It can help develop a deep understanding of what it means to be autistic and what it means to live with an autistic individual. However, a word of caution, it is essential to bear in mind that there is no such thing as 'one size fits all' in autism. Every autistic person is unique and will display and manage autistic traits differently from other autistic people, depending on their personality, upbringing and experiences. It is important for a counsellor with personal experience of autism not to allow their own experience to bias their opinions or perceptions of the clients they are working with. This is especially true if the counsellor's experience was mainly negative.

Many factors will affect how an autistic adult manages their relationships; one particularly important factor is their childhood and upbringing. Nurture plays a vital role in the development of all children, regardless of whether the child is autistic. Upbringing and childhood experiences can greatly impact how an individual manages relationships in adulthood. One autistic gentleman described his upbringing as an only child as completely solitary; he was home-schooled and, except for some distant cousins, hardly had the chance to interact or play with other children. This upbringing protected him from the anxiety caused by attending a chaotic school environment and having to socialize and interact with others, but it did not prepare him for work, society, friendships and relationships in later life. The difficulties this gentleman faced in forming and maintaining relationships were very different to those of another individual who had benefited from early recognition of autism and been taught coping strategies to control and reduce the anxiety that being in a social environment caused.

An individual's attachment style will also be affected by their upbringing, and this applies equally to both partners. However, autistic traits can sometimes mimic particular attachment styles, and it can prove difficult on first meeting to decipher what is due to autism and what is due to attachment style. This will take time and rely heavily on the counsellor's experience and knowledge.

We would advise that any decision to work with autistic individuals or couples should be first discussed in supervision, as having a supervisor who understands the unique nature of autism and neurodiverse relationships will also be important. If a counsellor finds their present supervisor is not experienced in this area, then seeking out a supervisor who might be more knowledgeable would be beneficial. If the counsellor is reluctant to change supervisors, then maybe explore arranging an external supervisor with knowledge of autism who can be called on when needed.

BEING CONGRUENT WITH CLIENTS

Being congruent and honest with clients paves the way for a trusting and secure therapeutic relationship. This information is usually supplied in the professional profile that a counsellor would use for advertising and that clients are provided with prior to arranging their first session. A counsellor should consider what would be helpful for their clients to know. It would be useful for clients to know whether a counsellor has personal experience of living with an autistic individual, whether that be a parent, sibling, child or partner. Equally, it would be relevant to disclose if the counsellor is also autistic or neurodivergent. Information such as this would be important to disclose before or during the first session. Leaving this until later in the therapeutic process could cause mistrust or uncertainty.

Clarification regarding the experience of autism is important, but also understanding the challenges of being autistic can be very relevant for the non-autistic partner. If the counsellor is autistic, then it would be important to reassure the couple that there is an adequate understanding of the non-autistic partner's experience and the issues they may be dealing with.

Other relevant information is the training and experience that a counsellor has undertaken or gained. Neurodiverse autistic couples coming for counselling will need to be reassured that they are in safe hands and that the counsellor they are trusting with their relationship will give it the time, respect and care that it deserves.

If the counsellor works within an agency, little information on the counsellor's experience, training or whether they are neurodiverse is offered. Counsellors are often allocated to clients rather than clients choosing the counsellor. This is something that we believe is long overdue for change. If an individual needed to see a specialist for a specific condition, then, unless paying privately, they would be allocated a specialist in the UK by the National Health Service. They would be provided with the name of the specialist they had an appointment with beforehand. They would be able to research that specialist and check out their qualifications. It makes sense that the same should be offered through counselling agencies. This would reassure the couple and, for the autistic partner, remove some of the ambiguity surrounding the meeting.

CONSIDER THE TIMINGS OF SESSIONS

Most counselling sessions are limited to 50 minutes. This is often not enough when a counsellor is working with a neurodiverse couple, as an autistic individual can require longer to process information, especially if that information is emotionally demanding. We would recommend sessions lasting 90 minutes or more. The first session in particular would ideally be at least 90 minutes as it is an important assessment. We know this may not be possible for some organizations, but for counsellors working in the private sector, it is an important detail to consider.

One factor that should be considered when working for longer session times is the importance of self-care by the counsellor. Working with an autistic neurodiverse couple will require developing a dualistic approach in the therapy provided. What works for the autistic client and what works for their non-autistic partner will be very different. The neurodiverse couple will both be processing information differently and have different sets of needs. A counsellor whose training is integrative can have an advantage here and may find that a cognitive behavioural therapy (CBT) approach will work best for the autistic client. In contrast, a more client-centred or emotion-focused approach will be more beneficial to the non-autistic client. Weaving two different approaches together can be tiring, especially when working sessions longer than 90 minutes.

Consideration must be given to the timing of sessions that a counsellor books in. Working back-to-back with neurodiverse couples is not recommended and is best avoided. We would recommend at least a 30-minute break between sessions. An overworked and tired counsellor will have little to offer their clients. Keeping healthy and maintaining self-care is an ethical requirement, one that is there to protect not just the client but also the counsellor.

CONSIDER GATHERING INFORMATION BEFORE THE FIRST SESSION

Another helpful consideration would be for the counsellor to be aware before meeting the couple whether one partner is autistic. This could be checked out by sending the couple a questionnaire to complete prior to the session or exploring the possibility on the telephone or via email before the initial session. The information may be freely given if there is a diagnosis or strong suspicion that one partner is autistic. This information being available beforehand will be very useful for the counsellor and give time to prepare and focus. However, the couple does not have to share this information prior to the first appointment.

It would prove equally helpful to have prior knowledge of whether the couple experience alexithymia or any other neurodiversity such as dyslexia, ADHD, dyspraxia or Tourette's syndrome.

If the counsellor has been informed that one or both partners is autistic, it would be beneficial to send photographs of the counselling room, waiting room and entrance to the building before the meeting. A professional photograph of the counsellor could also be helpful in reducing any pre-counselling anxiety for the autistic client. Going into a new environment without any information can feel particularly intimidating for the autistic partner, and having a visual picture of what to expect can work well in reducing anxiety and stress. Creating an environment that is calm and feels safe for the client is essential in all cases but is even more essential if the client is autistic.

It might be worth checking if there are sensory issues which should be considered. Even something like a picture hung out of alignment can distract an autistic client, as can the ticking of a clock or bright or fluorescent lighting. Checking in advance or with the couple during the first session can help set the scene for developing trust and creating a secure therapeutic alliance. Giving time to consider the environment and sharing this with the clients can indicate that the counsellor understands autism and the difficulties that sensory overload can cause. Where possible, using and remaining in the same room throughout therapy can also be very beneficial. If a room change is unavoidable, the counsellor should ensure that the client is given prior notice of this, as an unexpected change could increase anxiety and negatively impact the smooth running of the session.

GIVE CONSIDERATION TO FEELING PREPARED AND WELL-EQUIPPED BEFORE THE FIRST SESSION

A counsellor must ensure that they feel fully prepared and have the necessary paperwork, handouts and information before the first session. Autistic individuals are frequently visual learners and benefit greatly from having information written down. Ensure that a flip chart and pens are readily available in the counselling room. The counsellor could have an up-to-date reading list, information on being in a neurodiverse relationship and a resource list; these can all be very useful handouts for the couple. The autistic partner may benefit from being provided with a notepad and pen or being asked to bring one so that they can take notes if they wish. Others might ask if they can have a recording of the session;

this is something that would need to be decided by the counsellor, as taping a session might feel quite inhibiting for some. However, there are advantages to replaying the session, such as refreshing their memory and a more accurate recall of explanations and suggestions.

It is better to consider and be prepared for all eventualities and have the tools you need to hand. Although it is best to gather as much information as possible before the first session, this is not always achievable. The counsellor might discover in the first session that there is also the possibility or suspicion that alexithymia, dyslexia, dyspraxia or ADHD need to be considered. All these conditions are more likely to present themselves alongside autism than in the non-autistic population.

For a counsellor to work with autism, they should also understand other neurodiverse conditions and be able to offer the clients the reassurance that they need to feel understood and that they are in capable hands. Chapter 16 discusses this in more detail. Having information sheets on these conditions might prove useful and beneficial for both partners.

In conclusion, to offer autistic neurodiverse couples the best possible support and care, counsellors need to consider whether they have adequate experience and training to work in this area. If unsure, a counsellor should enhance their expertise by attending training sessions and developing their understanding and confidence in working with neurodiversity. Once this is achieved, the counsellor can go forward and arrange the first session working with neurodiverse couples. Hopefully, this will be the beginning of building strong and positive therapeutic relationships with many more neurodiverse couples in the future.

CHAPTER 18

The First Session

As with any relationship, building a therapeutic relationship based on trust and respect will take time and will not be achieved in the first session with the couple. However, the first session with a neurodiverse couple will be key in predicting the consequential stability and success of the therapeutic relationship that follows (Javier del Rio Olvera et al., 2022).

The aim of the first session is for the counsellor to:

1. Formulate an accurate picture of the relationship and both partners.

2. Reflect on what is being observed to the couple and illustrate an understanding of both perspectives.

3. Explore with each partner their expectations and the goals they want to achieve from the couple counselling.

4. Explain precisely what is realistically achievable.

5. Talk about considerations for online counselling.

6. Discuss what techniques and strategies will be implemented.

7. Give the couple a technique or exercise they can work on before the next session.

8. Summarize and write down the relevant points of the session and encourage the autistic partner to make notes.

9. Suggest an individual session for both partners if it would be beneficial. Be precise on the boundaries and confidentiality of these sessions.

FORMULATING AN ACCURATE PICTURE OF THE RELATIONSHIP AND BOTH PARTNERS

The reason the majority of couples decide to seek support from relationship counselling is the ongoing conflict they are experiencing between them and a failure to resolve their issues alone. The effect of this conflict might be expected to impact both partners equally, with them both presenting in the session as being stressed, anxious or frustrated by each other. In our experience, this is rarely the case when seeing a neurodiverse couple for the first time. This is particularly true when the non-autistic partner is female, regardless of whether the relationship is heterosexual or a lesbian relationship.

In our survey, we received reports from both the autistic and non-autistic partners that they felt the counsellor was biased and favoured the autistic partner in preference to the non-autistic partner. It appears from the survey that most of the counsellors working with the couples were non-autistic; this contradicts research that found non-autistic individuals are more likely to develop negative first impressions of autistic individuals compared to their non-autistic counterparts (Sasson et al., 2017). This bias is even more likely if the counsellor is unaware that the client is autistic.

For many of the respondents in our survey, it was often the case that the counsellor was unaware that one partner was autistic and yet still appeared to form a better therapeutic relationship with the autistic client than with their partner. There could be two reasons for this. First, it can appear on first impression that the non-autistic partner is the one displaying all the emotions, which can take the form of distress, frustration, anger and sometimes all three. It is likely that the non-autistic partner may have been trying for months or years to convince their partner that they should seek support from counselling, and it is also likely that by the time they get to the counselling room, they will be desperate to be believed and understood. They may expect that the counsellor will not just be empathetic to their situation and understand how they feel but will be able to explain to their partner why they are so upset. They may have also spent years suppressing their emotions as they realized displays of emotion only served to widen the gap between them and their autistic partner. Going to couple counselling can open the floodgates for all those emotions to come out and be heard.

This is in direct contrast to how the autistic partner will probably present, especially as they may have spent many years of their lives masking their feelings and autistic traits in a desperate attempt to appear 'normal'. The autistic partner is often likely to present in a couple counselling session as calm, polite and in control, which will be very different to their partner's experience of them in the safety of their home.

It would be easy for the counsellor to find the autistic client more approachable and easier to work with. The problem is that the counsellor is not seeing the reality of either partner as neither will be presenting as their authentic self. The autistic partner is likely masking and suppressing emotions of stress and anxiety, while the non-autistic partner is in emotional overload brought on by a desperate attempt to be heard and believed by the counsellor. It would be all but impossible for any counsellor to form a positive and congruent therapeutic relationship that would remain stable if the counsellor is not given an accurate picture of the relationship the couple shares.

It will not always be the case that a neurodiverse couple presents in this way, and the best scenario for counselling would be that the couple and counsellor are already aware that one partner is autistic or that the couple strongly suspect that this is the case. However, it appears from the reports in the survey that this knowledge also caused a bias in the counselling room. This was described by an autistic female partner in the survey, reporting that she felt all the counsellor's attention was focused on her and her autism, and her non-autistic partner's needs were totally disregarded.

Once again, the counsellor will need to ensure that having the knowledge that one partner is autistic does not cause their attention to become focused on the autistic partner alone. This could impact both partners in a negative way, leaving the autistic partner to feel they are the reason for the problems and the non-autistic partner feeling their needs are being neglected and marginalized by the counsellor.

For a counsellor, at this initial stage in the therapeutic relationship, showing that they have a deep understanding of the long-term effects of being a neurodiverse couple is paramount to the success and outcome of the couple therapy.

REFLECTING BACK TO THE COUPLE WHAT IS BEING OBSERVED ILLUSTRATES AN UNDERSTANDING OF BOTH PERSPECTIVES

The counsellor will need to reflect back to the couple what is being observed and reassure both partners that they understand how difficult it is for each of them. This reflection should be addressed to each partner separately, as each must feel understood differently.

The autistic partner will need to know that the counsellor has a thorough understanding of what being autistic means in a relationship. They will need acknowledgement from the counsellor that they are aware of the issues they face. For example, managing confrontation, working out what their partner wants and needs from them, dealing with the expectations that they can offer spontaneous empathy in confusing emotional situations and, for some, sadly, managing the feelings of failure in the relationship. All these feelings are unlikely to be openly expressed, especially if the autistic partner also experiences alexithymia. The counsellor will need to discuss with the autistic partner the implications of masking and enquire whether this applies to them. If so, the counsellor should acknowledge this and share that the mask will hopefully no longer be necessary as trust builds.

The non-autistic partner will need to know that the counsellor is aware that being in a neurodiverse relationship can be difficult. It is unlikely that their partner will have been able to meet their emotional needs, and this will particularly be the case if there was no awareness of autism (at all, or for a period of time earlier in the relationship). Be sure to add that although it was never their partner's intention not to meet their needs, that does not negate the feelings of emotional deprivation they are experiencing. Reassure the non-autistic partner that their feelings of loneliness, frustration and maybe anger can be alleviated with the right approach and self-care.

How the counsellor handles this will set the tone for the remainder of the therapeutic relationship and increase the likelihood that the couple will return. Our research showed that the most important variable in the outcome of counselling was how the counsellor understood each partner's feelings. The first step towards building a trusting therapeutic relationship should be taken in the first session with the counsellor showing empathy and understanding; without these important attributes, trust and security in the counselling relationship will not be developed.

EXPLORE WITH EACH PARTNER THEIR EXPECTATIONS
AND THE GOALS THEY WOULD LIKE TO ACHIEVE
FROM THE COUPLE COUNSELLING

This exploration could be done in the form of a question, or it could be part of a written exercise. If the exploration is spoken, the counsellor must ensure that the question is understood. We would recommend addressing any questions regarding the couple's relationship with the autistic partner first. Doing this will avoid the risk that the autistic partner will simply echo the reply from their partner. This is not due to trying to deceive or belittle. It is due to the fear of saying the wrong thing and a way to avoid the possibility of any confrontation. This is a pattern of behaviour which we have observed many times in autistic partners, who have discovered in the past that they can unintentionally give the wrong reply and cause their partner to become upset or angry.

Although the best way to gain insight into what the autistic partner really wants and needs is to ask them any questions first, it may not always feel like the right time to do so. If, at this initial stage of the counselling, it might feel too stressful for them, then another way is to have a prepared questionnaire sheet and ask each of them to fill it out. The counsellor can then decide whether to read the answers out loud or give a brief and safe summary of what the couple are both hoping to gain from counselling. We have found that autistic partners often reply to this question saying they just want to know how to make their partner happy and hope the counsellor will tell them how to achieve this (Aston, 2012, p. 18).

What the couple want to achieve from counselling will vary greatly between couples, and this will affect how the counselling process is determined. Sometimes, a couple will attend counselling because one or both partners wish to end the relationship and would like support in achieving this. We will discuss breakups and divorce in more detail in Chapter 22. At times, the conflicts within the relationship may not have any relevance as to whether the couple are neurodiverse. Substance abuse, alcoholism and addictive behaviours such as pornography addiction and computer gaming can occur in any relationship. However, the way they are managed and resolved will be different if autism is in the equation. It may be more appropriate and beneficial for the counsellor to refer the partner for individual therapy to a counsellor who understands autism and specializes in that particular field.

EXPLAIN PRECISELY WHAT IS REALISTICALLY ACHIEVABLE

The aim of couple counselling is to empower both partners to achieve personal growth, understand their differences, have realistic expectations and manage and resolve the difficulties and problems they may face in the future. At no time should counselling encourage dependency; what the couple achieve will be their achievements, not the counsellor's. The counsellor's role when working with an autistic neurodiverse couple is to be an educator, translator and guide. Initially, as a guide, the counsellor will be leading the couple, then next walking alongside the couple, and finally walking behind the couple. It can be useful to describe this analogy to clients: counselling is a journey, and for many couples, it will be one of the most important journeys they make because its outcome may affect not just the couple's future but the future lives of their children, grandchildren and all who are close to them.

Counselling cannot change a neurodiverse couple into a neurotypical couple. Sometimes the non-autistic partner can hope and expect that counselling will somehow teach their partner to be non-autistic. It is important for the counsellor to explain from the outset that autism is not something to be 'cured'. There can be adjustments and the capacity to learn better ways of communication, but the fundamental neurological difference between the couple and how their brains are wired will always exist. Counselling can offer the tools required to overcome the differences and make the relationship manageable, but only the couple can decide whether or not they put them to use.

CONSIDERATIONS FOR ONLINE COUNSELLING

If the relationship counselling is taking place online it is very relevant for the counsellor to be aware that the autistic client's facial expressions may not indicate their level of stress or anxiety and how they are feeling. It may be difficult for the counsellor to gauge what is going on for their client and asking them may not always provide an accurate answer, especially if alexithymia is present. From the outset there will need to be an agreement between client and counsellor regarding how they might communicate their stress level. For example, colours or numbers. This could be verbally or on a chart.

As with face-to-face counselling, autistic clients should be informed that they do not need to make eye contact, if doing so makes them feel uncomfortable or inhibits their ability to focus. In addition, it is not uncommon for autistic individuals to be affected by visual sensory sensitivities and these can be experienced as uncomfortable and sometimes painful. The autistic client may ask if they can wear sunglasses or to look away from the screen or turn the lights down. This should be encouraged as it will greatly reduce the level of anxiety that the autistic client may be experiencing. The counsellor should enquire as well whether it would be of benefit for the autistic client if they were to turn their lights down or not look directly at the screen.

DISCUSS WHAT TECHNIQUES AND STRATEGIES WILL BE EXERCISED

For the first session, it will not be possible to determine exactly what techniques and strategies will work for each couple, and much will be down to trial and error. At this stage in the therapeutic relationship, it is important to reassure the autistic partner that they will not be given any exercises that are outside their remit. Establish that all exercises and strategies will be explained beforehand, and there will be no sudden surprises. All instructions will be made clear and written down in advance.

Ensure both partners that they will be respected for their differences and that not all techniques and exercises will be applied to both. Each partner has a different set of needs and different requirements. The counsellor will be a translator and mediator between them, teaching them better ways to communicate and interact, and helping the couple to develop realistic expectations of what each can consistently achieve as a partner and contribute to the relationship.

GIVE THE COUPLE AN EXERCISE THEY CAN WORK ON BEFORE THE NEXT SESSION

Giving the couple a simple exercise they can work on before their next appointment can prove very beneficial to the counselling process. This should be something positive and non-confrontational. It could be to consider two qualities their partner brings to the relationship or what they like most about their partner. The exercise might be based on something that was raised in the session. It will be for the counsellor to determine for each couple; it is also a good plan to have something in mind. Whatever is given, it is important that the exercise is written down to ensure that it is understood.

SUMMARIZE AND WRITE DOWN THE RELEVANT POINTS OF THE SESSION AND ENCOURAGE THE AUTISTIC PARTNER TO MAKE NOTES

Some of the autistic respondents in our survey raised the need for instructions and summaries to be written down or for them to be allowed to take notes throughout the session. Autistic individuals often tend to be visual learners, and having relevant details written down can help alleviate the stress and pressure of remembering what often feels like a stressful or emotional situation.

Summarizing and writing notes can take time, which is one of the reasons why longer sessions are even more advisable. We recommend formulating a summary of the session for the last 10 to 15 minutes before it concludes. We recommend that the couple be involved in its construction. The couple could be given the summary, or the counsellor could take a copy and email it to both partners with their consent.

SUGGEST AN INDIVIDUAL SESSION FOR BOTH PARTNERS IF FELT IT WOULD BE BENEFICIAL. BE PRECISE ON THE BOUNDARIES AND CONFIDENTIALITY

If, during or at the end of the first session, the counsellor feels that it would be beneficial to have an individual session with both partners, then this should be offered to the couple to decide in the session or to take some time to consider. The counsellor should explain that the purpose of the individual session is to allow time for each to put forward their own perspective and relationship needs so that a better understanding of both partners and their relationship can be developed. It is equally important that before the individual sessions, the counsellor explains in detail the level of confidentiality and the boundaries that need to be put into place.

It would be unethical for the counsellor to keep secrets or to know something that affects the relationship and keep it from the other partner. We recommend that a statement on this be written down, and each partner then signs their agreement that they give the counsellor permission to reveal any secrets to the other partner so that counselling can continue. For example, if one partner were to inform the counsellor that they were having an affair without the others' knowledge, it would be unethical to collaborate with the partner in keeping this secret.

If a secret is disclosed, the counsellor should first encourage the partner to share 'the secret' with their partner themselves before the next session, or to be aware that the counsellor will reveal this at the beginning of the session. Maintaining the trust of both partners in couple counselling is vital to fulfilling the principle ethical guidelines laid down by all governing bodies. If, however, is the counsellor considers that revealing 'the secret' would put either partner at risk, then we recommend that a supervision session be arranged immediately to discuss the issues and decide on a course of action.

REFERENCES

Aston, M. (2012). *What men with Asperger syndrome want to know about women, dating and relationships*. Jessica Kingsley Publishers.

Javier del Rio Olvera, F., Rodriguez-Mora, A., Senin-Calderon, C., & Rodriguez-Testal, J. F. (2022). The first session is the one that counts: An exploratory study of the therapeutic alliance. *Frontiers in Psychology, 13.* https://doi.org/10.3389/fpsyg.2022.1016963

Sasson, N., Faso, D., Nugent, J., Lovell, S., Kennedy, D. P., & Grossman, R. B. (2017). Neurotypical peers are less willing to interact with those with autism based on thin slice judgments. *Scientific Reports, 7,* 40700. https://doi.org/10.1038/srep40700

CHAPTER 19

Working with Autistic Neurodiverse Couples

In our survey we asked respondents if they were aware of the modality their counsellor was trained in and what type of therapy they were offered. The answers to this question covered a whole range of talking therapies, including psychodynamic, CBT, Gestalt, person-centred, relation-trained and many others. It is interesting that we found no correlation between the type of therapy offered and the level of satisfaction in the counselling. The only link we found was that seeing a counsellor who was experienced and knowledgeable in autism or trained to work with autistic neurodiverse couples resulted in a higher rate of overall satisfaction with the counselling the couples received. These couples reported a more trusting and secure therapeutic relationship with a more positive and satisfying outcome from the therapy they had received.

This strongly suggests that knowledge and training in understanding autism and how this affects both the autistic and the non-autistic partner is paramount to the success of the counselling. It will be important that a counsellor adapt the way they work to benefit the two very different needs of the couple they are working with. No two people in a relationship are alike, and their needs will be different; however, for an autistic partner and a non-autistic partner in a relationship, the gap between them will be far wider, and in many cases counselling alone will not be able to bridge this gap. The aim of the counselling should be to find a satisfactory compromise that will keep the relationship healthy and realistically positive.

The focus of counselling will be on accepting the differences, understanding the differences and being very reasonable about what is achievable. Counselling will need to take on a dualistic approach to address the different needs of the couple, combining a basic CBT/solution-focused approach for the autistic partner with a more client-centred and emotion-led approach for the non-autistic partner. Having some training in both these areas will be an advantage to the counsellor.

To some counsellors, the prospect of working this way can seem daunting, and they may make the decision not to work with neurodiverse couples, a decision which should be respected. For others, though, working with autism can hold a strong appeal, and this is often due to the counsellor having personal experience with autism and an eagerness to support others in a similar situation. These counsellors have a huge advantage in that they already have knowledge of what it means to be autistic, and this, in many cases, removes the uncertainty and reservations that might undermine the counsellor's confidence in working in this area.

All couples seeking counselling will be attending for different reasons. Some will already be aware that one partner is autistic, whereas others will be uncertain or will be coming for counselling to explore that idea. The one issue that will present itself in almost all cases is the struggle for communication between partners. Improving communication and explaining the double empathy problem will be the primary focus of the counselling, and finding ways to make this easier and more available to the couple will be a key task for the counsellor.

In addition to communication, there may be issues over socializing, balancing daily tasks, responsibilities, quality time together and childcare. In addition, for the non-autistic partner, issues regarding emotional neglect, self-doubt and self-neglect will need to be addressed by the counsellor. Infidelity does occur in neurodiverse relationships, but we have found it is less likely than in the general population, especially among autistic men. Sometimes, though, it can feel for non-autistic women that their autistic partner is having another relationship with their work or special interest. This is where finding a satisfactory balance for both partners is important.

It is important when working with an autistic partner that the boundaries of the therapeutic relationship are made very clear from the outset and put into writing for the client to read and understand. These boundaries would be very similar to the boundaries set up for all clients and would cover appointment timings, cancellations, contact, safeguarding and confidentiality. The difference here is that it would be beneficial to go through this in detail with the autistic client to check it is fully understood and agreed to. It is important to never presume when working with neurodiversity that something has automatically been understood.

WHAT DO THE COUPLE HOPE TO GAIN FROM COUNSELLING?

A clear picture of what the couple are hoping to achieve from counselling needs to be discussed and clarified. It can help the couple and, in particular, the autistic partner to come prepared for this question. Giving prior notice of this and asking the couple to make a list of goals before the session can give the autistic partner time to consider and consolidate their list. Hopefully, the couple will have discussed their hopes and goals together beforehand, and both their goals will be somewhat similar. This can make it far more straightforward for the counsellor to plan the work to be done.

Unfortunately, though, we have found that having similar lists of goals is often not the case with a neurodiverse couple, especially if communication between them has totally broken down. We have both learnt to be prepared for the unexpected in our work. For example, a non-autistic partner might ask the counsellor to tell their autistic partner that they are divorcing them. The autistic partner in contrast might be unaware that there is any major issue or problem in the relationship. This unawareness could be due to difficulties in reading their partner's non-verbal body language or being too preoccupied with their interest or work to notice. Equally, it might be an autistic partner asking the counsellor to tell their partner that they can no longer tolerate the noise they make when breathing at night or eating a meal. They may go on to announce that they no longer wish to share the bedroom or eat with them. This may come as a total surprise to the non-autistic partner, who may question why this has not been mentioned before. It is not unusual for the autistic partner to remain silent over issues that trouble them, and this is nearly always due to fear of confrontation and criticism. Their hope is that the counsellor will understand and be able to explain to their partner, without any conflict, the reasons for this.

The raising of these issues can trigger many suppressed emotions and the counsellor may need to calm the situation down and possibly arrange for the next sessions to be individual sessions. This will allow both partners the space and safety to raise their concerns and talk them through with the counsellor. If this is the case the counsellor must be sure that rules regarding confidentiality are understood.

ASSESSING THE COUPLE'S RELATIONSHIP

Using self-assessment questionnaires (Aston, 2021) can prove invaluable as a way to gain insight into the perceptions of both partners on their feelings and where they feel they stand in the couple's relationship. These questionnaires can be specifically modified to suit the couple the counsellor is working with. They do not rely on words for answers, which can remove the stress and anxiety caused when asking autistic individuals to find the right descriptive word to describe how they feel, due to alexithymia. The questionnaires use numbers to express the level of affect each question has. For example, for the question 'I am satisfied with our sexual relationship', the answers would be on a numeric scale of 0 to 10 and the respondent would simply circle which number they believe describes them. The same questionnaires are given to each partner for them to complete individually and then handed back to the counsellor who can share with the couple the results and especially the differences in the answers. For example, if in answer to the question 'I am satisfied with our sexual relationship', one partner circled nine and the other two, then this would be an area to explore further and discuss. The answers to the questionnaire can allow the counsellor to put together a plan for the sessions as they will highlight the areas that need working on and the areas that are going well between them. These assessment questionnaires are also useful for reapplying in review sessions so that the counsellor can monitor both negative and positive improvements and changes in the relationship.

EDUCATION: WHAT IS AUTISM, AND WHAT IS NOT?

Education and the need for explanation and understanding were mentioned frequently in our survey. What traits are due to a partner being autistic and what are due to personality or past experience can seem very confusing for the non-autistic partner and sometimes the autistic partner, too. What makes this more confusing is the autistic partner's ability to mask. Masking or camouflaging autistic traits is achievable by the majority of autistic individuals, particularly when trying to form an intimate relationship.

Masking, though, can give the non-autistic partner a false sense of security and an unrealistic view of what is actually achievable and maintainable in the relationship. Masking increases the non-autistic partner's expectations of their partner, so confusion and disillusionment take over when the mask inevitably comes off over time. This is further exacerbated by the fact that the autistic partner will possibly continue the masking with friends and at work, leaving the non-autistic partner even more confused and more likely to believe that the problems are all personal to them. Relationship counselling will need to educate both partners on this and help the non-autistic partner build a realistic picture of what is healthily achievable in the relationship. Aiding the couple in developing a true understanding of what can and cannot be changed in the long term can be a relief for both partners and create realistic expectations while taking the pressure off the autistic partner to deliver and maintain the unachievable.

COMMUNICATION

Working on communication between the couple will be ongoing throughout all sessions. The counsellor will be working as a translator. It is said that being in a neurodiverse relationship means talking in two different languages. Sometimes, misinterpretation in communication will be subtle, and there will be little to show that the message has not been understood. The counsellor will need to be very alert and observant in spotting this and very quick to press the 'pause button' in the session. For example, one couple were having a heated discussion in the counselling session regarding the amount of time the autistic partner spent pursuing his interest in sailing. His non-autistic partner was very upset saying she had arranged for them to take the children to visit her parents, as her mother had been unwell and was unable to travel to them. Her partner had not mentioned to her till the last minute that he had entered a sailing competition and would not be able to join them. She felt let down, unsupported and very angry. In the middle of her argument with him, she said, 'I am fed up with being at the bottom of your priority list, and if you don't care about me, then you should leave, and then you could go sailing every day'. Her argument continued. Although there was no obvious reaction from the autistic partner, the counsellor put up her hand and said, 'Can we just pause here, as I would like to ask your husband what he just heard you say?' To which he replied that his wife had just said that he had to leave as she did not want him there any more. This was the only component of what his wife had said that he recalled, and he had totally missed his wife's true intent. Leaving was the last thing she wanted him to do; she wanted him to apologize and tell her he did care about her and how important his family was to him. She missed him because he was away from home all the time and hoped he would realize how upset and neglected this made her feel. Basically, she was seeking affirmation that he loved her more than his sailing.

It is very important for a counsellor, when working with autistic neurodiverse couples, to pay close attention to what is being said and how it is likely to be interpreted by the listener. Without this focus and attention by the counsellor, important information could be overlooked and one partner may presume it was heard as intended. The double empathy problem will cause both partners to struggle in accurately reading the feelings and intentions of the other and neither partner can presume their assumptions of the other are correct. Accurate interpretation can never be presumed in a neurodiverse couple as both partners are talking in different languages. The counsellor will need not just to understand the language of both partners, but also be able to understand how, sometimes, what is heard can be selective, especially by the autistic individual. If the conversation is emotional or the autistic individual believes they are 'under attack' what is heard can be selective and taken out of context. This has been described as 'not seeing the wood for the trees'. It is due to information overload. Pressing the pause button will slow things down and give the autistic partner time to process and explain what they have heard. It will also allow the counsellor to consider and rephrase the dialogue in a way that can be correctly understood. This will also teach the couple how easy it is for words and their real intent to be misunderstood.

Both partners will have a preferred and very different way of expressing how they feel. The autistic partner will require that communication be clear, direct, logical and totally unambiguous, in contrast to the non-autistic partner, whose communication may contain much emotional expression, double meanings, ambiguous references, sarcasm and innuendos that would be understood by the counsellor but not their partner. When the counsellor pauses the session, they need to check what has been heard or intended from each partner and just how much of the communication has been correctly understood.

One of the main gains from doing this is that it will also show each partner how much of their communication is being misinterpreted, and they will be learning from the counsellor the importance of reviewing and reframing what they have said into a language that both understand. This can make a very positive change in the relationship and aid the couple to gain a better insight into each other. It can help to name this as 'Pressing the pause button' or if the moment has passed then 'Rewinding the tape'. Using these inoffensive phrases can teach the couple to do the same with each other when they are unsure that their communication has been understood.

UNDERSTANDING WHAT HAS BEEN SAID BY THE CLIENTS

Just as it is important to ensure that the couple understand each other, it is equally important for a counsellor to check that they understand the meaning behind what has been said to them. This particularly applies when listening to what the autistic partner has to say. Studies are now showing that non-autistic individuals are more likely to misunderstand autistic individuals than they are other non-autistic individuals (Milton, 2012). One of the reasons for this is that non-autistic individuals often rely on facial expressions, eye contact and body language. These are all aspects of communication that counsellors are often highly sensitive to and are tuned to pick up on. Just a shift in body language, such as suddenly folding one's arms, looking away, emphasizing a word, changing voice pitch, grimacing or even a slight smile, can replace a hundred spoken words in communication. A well-trained and experienced counsellor will be very advanced in this area. However, when it comes to reading autistic individuals, these valuable skills can be ineffective as autistic individuals do not always use these indicators to communicate their feelings or intent. Instead, an autistic individual may display misleading signals and often at the wrong time, such as smiling when the topic is woeful or suddenly raising their voice when there is no reason to do so. A counsellor will need to be very aware that this could be what is occurring in the room and check when possible that they have understood the content and intention of what has been said. Part of the counselling will also be to teach the non-autistic partner to do likewise.

EXPLORE EACH PARTNER'S LOVE LANGUAGE

Some respondents in the survey stated how the counsellor had discussed with them and explained what is meant by the five love languages, which was considered a positive in the counselling. The idea that every individual has a combination of five ways of expressing love and expecting love was first proposed by Gary Chapman in his ground-breaking book first published in 1992. His book proposes that an individual's love language can be categorized in five ways: words of affirmation, quality time, receiving gifts, acts of service and physical touch. Chapman states in his book that 'Your emotional love language and the language of your spouse may be as different as Chinese from English' (Chapman, 2015, p. 15).

This explanation was well received by the autistic partners, as it is applicable to all couples and does not feel as personal as something attributed purely to being autistic. There may be times when autism is simply suspected and not acknowledged, or the autistic partner would rather it was not investigated. Using this book can be very helpful in aiding such couples in working on their communication and making sense of the difficulties they are experiencing.

When explaining the concept of the five love languages, the counsellor needs to explain to the couple that individuals are unlikely to have just one love language but will offer and need a combination of the five. For example, a person might use 50% words, 30% acts of service and 20% gifts. The counsellor could, with the couple, put together pie charts to illustrate this for each partner, both on what they offer and also on what they require from each other, and then compare them together in the session. It is important to make visuals as much as possible for the autistic partner and to give them copies to take home, as autism is associated with greater abilities in visual rather than verbal conceptualization.

WORDS DO NOT WORK: FINDING ALTERNATIVE WAYS TO COMMUNICATE

Words and especially words for feelings can be difficult for the autistic partner, who, especially if alexithymia is present, may find having to describe inner emotions in words and participate in emotional conversation both tiring and taxing. The counsellor can explain this to the non-autistic partner by using the analogy of giving someone who has dyslexia multiple spelling tests. The dyslexic individual would soon feel tired and drained; having to use emotional expression to find words to describe innermost feelings is no different for someone who is autistic. Finding an alternative is essential for the counselling to be successful and for the couple to learn to communicate with each other. Words do not always work, and the more counselling uses different mediums for emotional communication, the better. Using the colour chart with number ratings to measure the intensity of the emotion (Aston, 2021), a wheel of emotions and typing using emails, text messages, poetry and music can all work well. Autistic individuals have been shown to have a great capacity to express some very deep and meaningful emotions when allowed to do so, using a medium of expression that works for them. An autistic individual who rarely told his partner he loved her was able to present her with a poem that brought tears to her eyes and gave her an insight into what lay beneath her partner's often cold and unemotional persona. An autistic concert pianist could express his love for his partner by the choice of music he played on the piano at home and the depth of feeling in how he interpreted the composition.

We cannot express enough the importance of the counsellor's role in allowing the autistic partner to find an alternative to using spoken words in a conversation to express thoughts and feelings.

THE SPECIAL INTEREST

Almost all autistic individuals have a special interest. This might be a hobby, a person (historical or contemporary), a pet or their work. Some interests can last a lifetime; others will have a use by date of hours to decades. To the autistic individual, their interest and the knowledge that is often acquired are, in many ways, fundamental to how that person is able to interact with others. It will be their area of expertise and a way to communicate and form friendships with like-minded individuals confidently. The counsellor will need to enquire about the special interest or interests and make use of this in the sessions. The interest is a way into the autistic individual's world, and using their interest to form analogies and metaphors to illustrate a point to the autistic partner can prove invaluable. The analogy used will obviously be dependent on the interest and will vary accordingly. Not all, but most interests require some kind of maintenance, research and effort, whether that be mechanical, renovating or body fitness. For example, if the interest was in vintage cars, forming an analogy between the importance of putting in effort to maintain and rebuild a car can be likened to the same amount of focus, effort and time required to maintain a healthy relationship.

Relationship counselling can also use the special interest to explain emotional/intangible feelings or needs in a tangible way that the autistic partner can relate to. For example, in one session with a neurodiverse couple, the non-autistic partner shared with the counsellor how low and alone she felt. She desperately needed more support, attention and care from her partner. The counsellor asked if she would compile a list of how her partner could achieve this. Her autistic partner read through the list, which included practical support and quality time, and he said that he understood what his partner was asking for and was happy to do these things.

When the counsellor reviewed the couple's progress a few weeks later, the non-autistic partner shared that her partner had only completed her list of requirements once. When asked about this, he replied that he had completed what was asked of him, and his partner had said she was happy about this, so why, as she was happy, would he need to do them again?

The counsellor was aware that the autistic partner was into gaming, and in one of the games he played regularly, his characters had a health bar that went from red (in distress) to green (healed). The counsellor asked the non-autistic partner to draw a health bar for herself, coloured it in red and green, and asked her to indicate where she felt she was on the health bar. She said she felt at the bottom of the red and that when he did things that showed her he cared, she would slowly move up towards the green. However, like his games, she would quickly slip back down into the red without reinforcement and topping up her health bar.

When it was explained in a tangible and visual way, with a metaphor relevant to his special interest, the autistic partner was able to have a much greater understanding of his wife's needs and how he could ensure that she stayed in the 'green' zone. The couple went on to use this as a way for the non-autistic partner to communicate when she needed his support. When she told him she was slipping into 'the red', he quickly understood what was needed and did not take it personally.

Relationship counselling can use special interests in many ways, such as explaining to one autistic partner who was into finance that helping with the house chores or putting the children to bed was like putting money into their partner's empty energy bank account.

For some couples, the interest may have been shared and will have been how they met. They may have shared the same course at university or been on a special interest holiday. More likely, it will have been within the working environment.

In the initial stages of the relationship, the autistic partner's intense knowledge of their interest may appeal to their new non-autistic partner, and they will be eager to share in the interest and participate if possible. However, as the relationship progresses, if the autistic partner's intensity in their chosen subject doesn't mellow, then this can become a bone of contention between the couple. The autistic partner will be left wondering why what used to be okay suddenly isn't, and the non-autistic partner may be left feeling neglected and at the bottom of their partner's priority list.

Relationship counselling will involve finding a compromise that works for both. What must be clear from the outset is that having a special interest is a central component of the personality of an autistic partner. It is vital for the autistic partner to be able to continue to maintain their interest for the sake of their mental health. The special interest offers the autistic partner both stress relief and emotional regulation by being a thought blocker for anxiety and depression and improving self-esteem and emotional resilience by acquiring knowledge and recognized expertise.

To disallow an autistic partner's special interest would be equivalent to disallowing the non-autistic partner's social support and connection with others—an analogy that may be appreciated by the non-autistic partner. Having said this, it is also important for the couple to share quality time dedicated to each other and the family. The counsellor will need to draw up ways and means of realistically building this into the relationship in a way that satisfies both and can be maintained. Drawing up a time plan together, bringing in some house rules and making time for each other will all need to be written down and agreed to. Using a big piece of flip chart paper for the couple to take home and put up on the wall can work well, as this will act as a reminder and give the couple something to refer back to.

MANAGING SENSORY ISSUES AND MELTDOWNS

We have already mentioned the importance of ensuring that the counselling room offers a safe and non-stimulating environment for the autistic partner to work in. This should also be considered within the couple's home environment.

Relationship counselling should discuss this with the couple and explore ways to improve the sensory environment at home for the autistic partner. If the space of the home allows it, having a safe and sensory calming place to retreat to can avoid meltdowns and decrease the risk of sensory overload.

This can be particularly relevant if there are children or teenagers in the family environment, as clutter, chaos and raised voices can become a daily occurrence. Having a stress-free, uncluttered place to retreat to for the autistic partner to calm and recharge can result in a more positive atmosphere for all concerned.

Rules concerning when and how this space is used will need to be discussed in the counselling session, and both parties will have to make compromises and agreements.

Obviously, space is not always available within the home, and other options will need to be considered. These could be an outside building, a place to sit in the garden, balcony or shed, or maybe just sitting in the car. Other alternatives for the autistic partner when feeling overloaded could be walking the dog, running or having some gaming time – the list is endless. These options will all need to be discussed and agreed upon together.

Sensory issues and sensory overload are very real and relevant issues that individuals with autism are expected to manage on a daily basis; they can be the cause of stress, anxiety, avoidance, frustration and meltdowns. Their effect on an individual and how they impact the couple's relationship can vary greatly between couples. We have found extreme variance between the individuals we have worked with, and there is no 'one size fits all' approach that can be recommended or applied here. The counsellor will need to explore this with the couple to draw together a plan of action that the couple can realistically work on.

SHARING RESPONSIBILITIES

For some couples, the issues they bring will weigh heavily on the imbalance of responsibilities shared between them, and this will need to be explored. It will often be the non-autistic partner, female or male, who will carry most of the responsibilities in the daily running and maintenance of the family. They may complain that despite the autistic partner working hard and providing an income, they are not communicating, participating or interacting with the family. The non-autistic partner may be left to deal with all the household chores, childcare, parent evenings, healthcare and social arrangements. This may be because they do not trust their partner to do it properly or because their partner does not want to be involved.

Relationship counselling will need to explore the reasons for this as they will be different for everyone. There can be many reasons why the autistic partner does not get involved in this way. Three such reasons are because the autistic partner:

1. has tried and got it wrong, so now avoids being involved altogether

2. has difficulty understanding the verbal instructions given, as they are often given in a chaotic environment and mixed in with a cocktail of messages

3. may get distracted and forget what they were supposed to do.

It may be one or all three of the above, or another reason; relationship counselling will need to investigate and ask questions to discover what is breaking down and what could be arranged to make it better.

Discussing the feasibility of having a weekly couple meeting can work well. This involves the couple putting aside time to sit down together for 30 minutes to an hour when they know they will not be interrupted. The counsellor should create a list of rules to achieve this that both partners agree to. This may include:

- turning off phones, the television, computers and the radio

- all children and pets being in bed, entertained or elsewhere

- both partners sending each other an agenda an hour before the meeting

- only including practical topics such as social arrangements, childcare and household tasks for the following week

- not including confrontational or emotionally charged topics

- allowing each other equal time to talk without interruption.

This list can, of course, be moderated to suit each couple in question.

It is very important that this is agreed upon equally by the couple and written down for them to take home and practice.

WHAT WORKS FOR YOUR CLIENTS AND WHAT DOES NOT – TASKS MUST BE DOABLE

Finding what works for the couple and what does not will be a matter of trial and error, and relationship counselling will be about experimenting and discovering what works for each couple.

Both the autistic and non-autistic respondents in the survey complained that the autistic partner was given exercises and expected to apply strategies that were totally outside their capacity. This led to the autistic partner feeling humiliated, frustrated and a failure. This goes against the very core of what relationship counselling should be aiming to achieve. It is highly likely that the counsellor did not understand autism and did not pick up on the signs that this was beyond the autistic partner's ability. However, rather than seeing this as an indication that something was amiss, it was interpreted as avoidance or a reluctance to try.

Tasks or exercises that are emotionally demanding on the autistic partner must be avoided. The counsellor should give time to assess what is doable and only use exercises that both clients are comfortable with.

In conclusion, the aim of couple counselling is to find a comfortable compromise which both partners can manage and from which the relationship can benefit. Working with autistic neurodiverse couples means working with differences. Both partners have different needs and will be processing information differently from each other. Both partners will have an equal right to be able to be who they are and have those needs met. Neither partner has the right to change or make their partner the same as them or sacrifice their needs to fit in. However, if these two very different people love each other and want to make a life together, they will have to find a compromise that works. The aim of counselling will be to find this place of compromise and realistic connection so that both partners can maintain their physical and mental health while enjoying the comfort of sharing their lives with the partner of their choice. Neurodiverse relationships can work and do, but not without commitment, education and understanding.

REFERENCES

Aston, M. (2021). *The autism couple's workbook* (2nd ed.). Jessica Kingsley Publishers.

Chapman, G. (2015). *The five languages of love that lasts*. Northfield Publishing.

Milton, D. E. M. (2012). On the ontological status of autism: The 'double empathy problem.' *Disability and Society, 27*(6), 883–887. https://doi.org/10.1080/09687599.2012.710008

CHAPTER 20

Barriers to Counselling

A study involving 300 couples in the general population explored the reasons for issues in couple counselling and discovered six distinct barriers. These were the cost of treatment, logistics, modality, trustworthiness, relational factors and a clear therapeutic process (Hubbard & Anderson, 2022). These barriers will apply to all couples attending relationship counselling regardless of whether they are neurodiverse. The aim of this chapter, though, is to focus on specific barriers that might be applicable to autistic neurodiverse couples.

EXERCISES

One barrier that showed itself to be quite relevant in our survey was the reports from respondents about the tasks and exercises they were given during the counselling process. Concerns were raised regarding the expectations from the counsellor that the couple would be able to complete exercises that were developed for non-autistic couples. In addition, the autistic partner was expected to be able to verbally express and communicate emotions and feelings, which put many under extreme pressure and stress. The consequence of this was a breakdown in the therapeutic relationship, as trust in the counsellor was broken, causing the autistic partner to shut down and often refuse to return to the relationship counselling. This had a very negative effect on the couple and frequently resulted in even more disharmony.

Autistic respondents to our survey frequently reported the difficulty they experienced when being given tasks and exercises that were inappropriate and emotionally demanding. The reasons they were given inappropriate tasks were due to both a lack of training and experience by the counsellor and a lack of awareness that their client was autistic and possibly alexithymic. Counsellors' lack of awareness, training and experience was the primary reason that relationship counselling failed according to our survey.

COMMUNICATION

Respondents to our survey expressed that they felt they and their partner were talking in different languages, and this is something that we have also found when working with couples. It is crucial that the counsellor can understand both languages and can work as a translator for the couple. The counsellor will need to be able to interpret the true intentions behind the words that the couple are trying to express.

Some couples might have a backlog of unresolved issues due to the many failed attempts to find a resolution through communication. Both will be exhausted and unlikely to have the energy to start learning a new way of communicating with their partner. Some may put all the blame on the other and expect that one partner should make all the effort and changes. This can prove challenging for the counsellor and a resolution may not always be achievable. The counsellor will require experience and much understanding to move the couple forward.

Alexithymia does not affect all autistic adults but has been found to affect a large percentage, and this can also be the reason for barriers in communication and counselling. Alexithymia will create an inability to find the right words to describe emotions, and only if this is understood by the relationship counsellor and the non-autistic partner will alternatives to verbal communication be accepted and put into place.

If the autistic partner is highly defensive and reacts negatively to any perceived criticism, the counsellor will need to handle the situation carefully. If this reaction extends to the counsellor as well as the non-autistic partner and cannot be resolved, it will restrict the communication and subjects that can be discussed safely in counselling. This will create barriers in communication, preventing the counsellor from moving the couple forward and generating positive change.

DENIAL OF BEING NEURODIVERSE

The second most common reason we found to be a primary barrier to success in counselling was denial and avoidance of accepting that the couple were neurodiverse. In some cases this was by the counsellor, and in others the autistic partner. Working with denial can be both exhausting for the counsellor and frustrating for the non-autistic partner. It can feel impossible to move the counselling forward, and it will feel like there is a constant proverbial elephant in the room. Without a compromise of some type, relationship counselling will not be successful.

Sometimes, a compromise can be finding another word for the differences experienced between the couple. One autistic gentleman could manage his divergence by this being referred to as the gender difference between him and his wife. He had read the popular book *Why Men Don't Listen & Women Can't Read Maps* by Allan and Barbara Pease (2001) and firmly believed that it adequately described both himself and his wife.

This did work to a point, but it meant he did not take any responsibility for the difficulties in the marriage and why his wife was struggling with emotional deprivation. He blamed her need for emotional input on the fact that she was a woman, and justified that he rarely showed her affection or offered any terms of endearment based on the fact he was a man.

STRENGTH OF AUTISTIC TRAITS

Another barrier could depend on the strength of the autistic traits in the partner. There may come a point in the counselling when it becomes apparent that managing any form of change proves impossible for the autistic partner to achieve. A study found a negative correlation between the strength of autistic traits and the relationship satisfaction reported by non-autistic wives (Renty & Roeyers, 2007). However, a later study reported that when autistic traits were greater, relationship dissatisfaction was more often reported by the autistic partner rather than the non-autistic partner (Pollmann et al., 2010).

SENSORY SENSITIVITY

One of the characteristics of autism that might impact on the counselling process and become a barrier to counselling is the level of sensory sensitivity. We have found this to vary greatly in the individuals we have worked with, and it is important to explore this in relationship counselling. If sensory sensitivity is greatly impacted by the environment, it could prevent an autistic individual from attending counselling in the first place. This is something that is now possible to overcome by working with the couple online. However, the non-autistic partner is less likely to benefit from this way of working and individual person-to-person counselling should be offered to them. Sensory sensitivity could become a barrier to sex, as we discussed in Chapter 15. It could also be a reason for not wanting children or a barrier to the couple sharing a social life or even a meal together. If these are aspects of a relationship that are important to the non-autistic partner and would cause feelings of deprivation, then they may feel unable to continue in the relationship, and some very difficult decisions will need to be made.

TIMING

As in all areas of counselling, in order to achieve a successful outcome, the timing has to be right. In relationship counselling, this is particularly important as it involves two people, and although the timing might feel right for one partner, it may not necessarily be right for the other. The relationship counsellor may soon find that they are working with two agendas, which may not be prepared to meet in the middle and compromise. This is a barrier that it will not be possible to overcome unless something shifts and changes. We have only found that this happens when a formal diagnosis is received, and both can view their relationship through fresh eyes. Many of the misunderstandings and false assumptions that have formed between them will now make sense. The discovery that a partner is autistic can change everything and re-establish a new form of hope for the relationship to work. Timing, logistics, financial input and situational factors can also be barriers to counselling, regardless of whether a couple is neurodiverse.

HAVING AN AUTISTIC CHILD

One barrier to take into account when working with an autistic neurodiverse couple is whether they have children who are also autistic and the level of support they need. Family life may be taking a toll, and organizing care and looking after children's needs can be exhausting and stressful. The energy needed for working at and rebuilding a neurodiverse relationship may be in short supply and, due to the time involved and the financial cost, it may simply be put on the back burner and ignored until the couple feel that they have the energy and space to prioritize it.

SHORTAGE OF RELATIONSHIP COUNSELLORS

The present shortage of relationship counsellors and the high demand for this specialism have led to very high prices for this service. Hopefully, this will change in the future, and neurodiverse couples will be able to access affordable services. Many organizations that work with couples are now seeking training for their counsellors so that neurodiversity-aware counselling is becoming more available.

COMPATIBILITY OF THE PARTNERS

Not all the barriers to counselling are specific to autism. Sometimes, the couple is simply not compatible and does not share the same fundamental needs, beliefs, attitudes or interests that are required to hold a relationship together. If this is the case, it is important that the counsellor points this out to the couple. Knowing this can remove the guilt and sometimes the shame that couples describe feeling when the blame for the relationship breakdown is placed entirely on being a neurodiverse couple.

REFERENCES

Hubbard, A. K., & Anderson, J. R. (2022). Understanding barriers to couples' therapy. *Journal of Marital and Family Therapy, 48*(4), 1147–1162. https://doi.org/10.1111/jmft.12589

Pease, A., & Pease, B. (2001). *Why men don't listen & women can't read maps: How to spot the differences in the way men and women think.* Orion Books.

Pollmann, M. M. H., Finkenauer, C., & Begeer, S. (2010). Mediators of the link between autistic traits and relationship satisfaction in a non-clinical sample. *Journal of Autism and Developmental Disorders, 40*, 470–478. https://doi.org/10.1007/s10803-009-0888-z

Renty, J., & Roeyers, H. (2007). Individual and marital adaptation in men with autism spectrum disorder and their spouses: The role of social support and coping strategies. *Journal of Autism and Developmental Disorders, 37*(7), 1247–1255. https://doi.org/10.1007/s10803-006-0268-x

CHAPTER 21

Mediation Services

The principal focus and aim of our survey was to discover both the positives and negatives that autistic neurodiverse couples experienced from attending relationship counselling. The survey did not cover mediation services. However, two non-autistic respondents reported that they were moving on from counselling and hoped to attend mediation together. In both cases, the respondents had decided to separate and divorce. We have, therefore, decided to include a brief chapter on mediation services here.

Major couple agencies in the UK, such as Relate and Relationships Scotland, recognize the need to have, in addition to counsellors, trained mediators available for couples who decide to separate or divorce. Not all relationships can be fixed, and not all partners want to continue; sometimes the only way forward for a couple is to separate. This is not an easy decision to make and is not always a mutual one. Divorce can be a highly stressful time and comes at a large financial cost, especially if there are disagreements over financial arrangements and child custody. Mediation can ease both the stresses and costs that come with divorce, especially if the couple are finding it difficult to agree and reach a compromise that works for both of them. Mediation is there to help and guide couples in their decision making and agreements. This is particularly useful when there are children involved. In most cases, it is not the actual divorce that causes the majority of the suffering and distress to children; it is the disagreements, arguments and battles that occur between the two people they depend on most.

If one of the parents is autistic, we have found that it is more likely that it will have been the non-autistic partner who made the difficult decision to separate and divorce. One of the reasons for this is due to the autistic partner's need to maintain consistency and routine in their daily life. Avoidance of incurring any changes can be a part of being autistic.

We have observed both male and female autistic individuals being the victims of some very dysfunctional relationships and remaining within them. Some autistic adults appear to display a very high tolerance for abusive behaviour. One of the reasons for this is to avoid the changes and uncertainty that leaving would bring. Insistence on sameness is a trait that forms part of the diagnostic criteria for autism (American Psychiatric Association, 2022, p. 57, diagnostic criteria B2).

Not all relationships that end are abusive, and couples can fall out of love just as they can fall in love. One partner may have moved on and changed, whereas the other remained static. Sometimes, being in a neurodiverse relationship can prove too hard and unmanageable, especially for the non-autistic partner, and particularly if their emotional needs are not being met.

If the decision to separate is the non-autistic partner's, their autistic partner will likely struggle to come to terms with this reality and do everything within their power to continue the relationship and avoid the necessary change. Seeing this can be heartbreaking for children who will be torn between the two parents and may blame the partner who wishes to divorce for the anguish they are suffering and witnessing.

In addition to these difficulties, it is also likely that one of the children, or more, may also be autistic and equally struggling with the unavoidable changes that are threatening their lives. This can be an inhibitory factor in seeking separation.

So, what do mediators working with autistic neurodiverse couples and families need to be aware of to be able to offer the most beneficial service possible to the couple and their family? To answer this question, we have divided the key points into sections, starting with one of the most important and initial areas to consider: understanding the couple.

UNDERSTANDING AUTISM AND NEURODIVERSE COUPLES

For mediation to be beneficial and successful, it is vital, as it is for counselling, for the mediator to understand what it means to be autistic and what it means to be in a neurodiverse relationship. Without this understanding, both partners could be at risk of being misunderstood and having unrealistic expectations placed on them.

As both numbers of people diagnosed with autism and divorce rates continue to rise, neurodiverse couples will likely find their way into the mediation process. The main aim of mediation is to find a calm and less stressful way for a couple to negotiate together while being allowed to express both points of view. Mediation is also there for the children involved and to help the parents decide what is best for them. To achieve this, the mediator must thoroughly understand autism and personal or professional training and experience of what it means to be in a neurodiverse relationship. Whether mediation is being offered on a private basis or through an organization, training and education to develop a deeper understanding of autism should be sought after or offered. Divorce is a time of transition, uncertainty, insecurity and extreme stress. Both partners will need to feel heard and understood.

The mediator may need to use the support available to them when working with a neurodiverse couple and seek to increase their awareness of autism and how it affects both adults and children. This can be achieved by reading research articles and blogs, and watching webcasts on autism and neurodiverse relationships readily available on the internet.

ARE THE COUPLE AWARE THAT ONE OF THEM IS AUTISTIC?

It may be that there is already a diagnosis or an awareness that one of the partners/parents is autistic, and in many ways, that can make the mediation process better informed and straightforward. Sometimes, though, there is not an awareness, or there is only an unconfirmed suspicion. Raising the fact that one of the partners may be autistic can be particularly difficult at this time, and the suggestion is likely to be totally denied by the autistic partner, especially if there are children involved.

At this stage in the divorce procedure, much anxiety could surround the suggestion of being autistic, often due to the fear that it will threaten access to the children and could become a basis for losing custody altogether. This fear is not unfounded, and accounts from both autistic mothers and fathers are now appearing on the internet describing how they believe that they were discriminated against for being autistic.

Being autistic does not mean being a bad parent any more than being dyslexic or having ADHD. These neurological differences do not render an individual incapable of caring for and loving their children. However, they mean that support from professionals and family should be readily available to call on without judgement. Autistic parents have much to offer their children, especially in the case of any children who are also autistic. They will have a far better understanding of their autistic child's struggles with sensory overload, difficulties in forming friendships and their need to spend time with their special interest.

The mediator will need to give reassurance to the autistic parent that they will not be judged or penalized simply for being autistic.

WHAT IF THERE IS NO DIAGNOSIS AND THE AUTISTIC PARENT IS IN DENIAL?

It can prove quite difficult to work with a neurodiverse couple if the autistic parent does not wish to acknowledge or investigate whether they are autistic. This can be made especially difficult if the non-autistic parent is quite convinced that their partner is somewhere on the autism spectrum. This conflict of opinion between the two parents will need sensitive handling by the mediator.

A mediator's role is not to diagnose autism but to be aware of the possibility. If there is an autistic child, then it is possible that one of the parents is also autistic, and this should be considered within mediation. We recommend that the mediator work with the couple in the same way that they would if there was a diagnosis in place, using the same strategies and tools recommended in this book.

In these circumstances, the mediator should also be aware of the effect this denial could have on the non-autistic parent. Confusion, uncertainty and frustration will probably have been building up over a long period of time. Answers to questions will have been sought, especially if a child is diagnosed. The non-autistic parent may have felt initially that discovering autism would have been the answer to the confusion they experienced. If, though, refusal to seek the advice of a professional and a denial of autism continues within the relationship, this could eventually become the reason that separation felt like the only alternative left.

WORKING WITH DISHARMONY

If the divorce is particularly disharmonious, seeing the couple in separate rooms may be the less stressful alternative. The mediator may find that communication has totally broken down between the couple. If this is the case, talking through a mediator may be the only way left for the couple to communicate. The mediator will be acting as the translator between the two of them. Mediation should encourage the couple to find alternative ways to communicate together when seeking to reach agreements, maybe by email or text.

Helping the couple to reach agreements on boundaries and contact arrangements can, if the autistic partner is struggling to accept and come to terms with the separation, prove difficult to manage, and we have known rare instances of the non-autistic partner being stalked. Stalking does need to be taken very seriously and should not be tolerated under any circumstances. If the stalking behaviour persists, it should be reported to the police. If stalking is suspected of becoming an issue and raised in mediation, strict boundaries need to be discussed and put into place. Most importantly, the consequences of stalking need to be logically and very clearly explained to the autistic parent.

Once the autistic partner is aware of the consequences of stalking, then that reality can be enough to prevent the behaviour. It is rarely the autistic individual's intent to cause harm; they are seeking information, and the last thing they would want is to be approached by the law. The behaviour is more likely to be about the extreme difficulty in managing the unavoidable changes that separation causes and being able to accept that daily routines and family life are no longer the same.

MANAGING CHILDCARE ARRANGEMENTS BETWEEN THE COUPLE

During this time of transition, finding a secure base from which to arrange childcare is important. How this is dealt with will vary between families, and making suitable decisions over shared care can be a challenging compromise. Once a decision is reached, arrangements need to be kept as firmly as possible regarding time, place and the return of the children.

All times, dates and arrangements made during the session must be written down and agreed to by both parents. If, for any reason, these plans need to be changed, the autistic parent must be given as much advance warning as possible. Last-minute changes to arrangements could send both the autistic parent and any autistic children into chaos and risk a possible meltdown.

USING REMINDERS, WRITING ARRANGEMENTS DOWN AND LISTING CHILDCARE NEEDS

If the non-autistic parent managed most of the childcare while the relationship was ongoing, then adequate and clear instructions should be supplied to the autistic parent. When arranging custody of the children, concerns have been raised in mediation as to whether the autistic partner will remember and maintain the children's needs in a way that they are accustomed to. This could be a concern for both parents, and it would be beneficial for all if the details of exactly what is required are clearly written down beforehand.

These details would need to state times for meals or naps, a list of foods preferred and how they should be cooked, medications and dosage if necessary, and any other relevant details. The autistic parent could then set their phone or Alexa to remind them, especially if timekeeping, decision-making abilities, and a lack of organizational skills are difficult for the parent. These abilities are described as executive functioning, and research has confirmed an association between autism and executive functioning difficulties (Rosello et al., 2022, p. 117).

LOOKING AFTER THE CHILDREN'S NEEDS

Divorce is a difficult and fractious time for all the children concerned. However, due to the uncertainty and unavoidable changes involved, it can prove particularly difficult for autistic children. The mediator should encourage parents to keep their children informed about what is happening and why. Avoiding conflicting and confusing information is important, as this will only increase the insecurities already experienced. It is better for autistic children to be informed by both parents together to explain and discuss what is occurring and how it will affect them.

Autistic children will not express their feelings in the same way as non-autistic children and are unlikely to seek to discuss their feelings of loss with others. Parents need to be advised to find alternative ways for their autistic child to express how they feel. This may be through art or writing or often through their special interest. One young autistic boy collected Pokémon cards and accumulated a large collection of which he was very proud. He knew all the names of the characters and what each one represented. He used these characters to express how he felt when asked by displaying the Pokémon character card he most strongly related to at the time. This gave his parents an insight into how he was feeling, and they were able to respond accordingly. If it is thought that using the services of a child therapist who specializes in autism might benefit the child, and the child is willing, then mediation could help to arrange this.

Sensory issues can be greatly exacerbated by stress and increase the likelihood of meltdown, both for the autistic parent and even more so for the autistic child or children. Parents should notify the school of the changes that are occurring in the home so that adequate measures can be put into place, such as teachers being aware when the child needs access to a quiet place in times of feeling overwhelmed.

Autistic children are likely to seek solace in their special interests. Allowing the child to maintain and continue to enjoy these interests will be crucial to their well-being. If the separation involves having to spend time in two different locations, then, if possible, access to their special interests should be continued in both places.

The interest may be in computer gaming, and there may be different tolerances for gaming in the two locations. One parent may have strict rules, while the other has no restrictions. This can be a cause of friction between the parents.

Mediation should discuss with the parents the possibility of 'bird nesting'. Bird nesting has become the term used for co-parenting a child in their primary home to avoid extreme changes. This involves the parents taking turns to live in the house and care for the children. This way of managing autistic children, although it can be inconvenient for the parents and sometimes not possible, is proving to be the most successful way of avoiding undue stress for an autistic child. Part of the mediation process should focus on how the parents might arrange this and how they could manage and maintain this.

Making small changes as gradually as possible to reduce anxiety and always keeping the child clearly and fully informed as to what is happening can be of great benefit. Unexpected changes and conflicting information will not be helpful and could break trust.

It is important for mediation to ensure that the non-autistic children's needs are also not overlooked. Unlike their autistic sibling(s), there is likely to be the need to talk about and express the cocktail of mixed emotions they might be experiencing. Talking this over with a counsellor in the safety of child therapy is highly recommended, and mediation could help arrange this, if the parents agreed, for the child concerned.

Mediation is an excellent and valuable service that is in place for the children as well as the parents. Although often working with conflict, it can also be very rewarding, especially when it serves to find resolutions and reduce the anxiety that the family are experiencing. Working with autistic neurodiverse families requires a different approach as there will be different needs to take into account. If these families are to be adequately supported within the mediation process, then it is crucial for the mediator to be trained and experienced in working in this area. Being trained in neurodiversity can only serve to increase the mediator's confidence and reassure parents that the mediation offered will be of benefit to the whole family.

REFERENCES

American Psychiatric Association. (2022). *Diagnostic and statistical manual of mental disorders (DSM-5-TR)*. APA.

Rosello, R., Martinez-Raga, J., Mira, A., Carlos Pastor, J., Solmi, M., & Cortese, S. (2022). Cognitive, social, and behavioral manifestations of the co-occurrence of autism spectrum disorder and attention-deficit/hyperactivity disorder: A systematic review. *Autism, 26*, 743–760.

CHAPTER 22

Endings

In counselling, endings are as important as beginnings. The first session can set the scene for how the counselling will proceed and how successful the therapeutic relationship will be, as we discussed in Chapter 18. Likewise, endings are what the clients are left with and take forward with them into the future. The couple will be putting into practice the learning skills and strategies that counselling will hopefully equip them with. Some describe this as handing clients a toolbox full of tools they can pull out and use when needed.

Sometimes, clients have asked how we will all know when the counselling is reaching fruition and coming to an end. We have described how, in most cases, it can become apparent by the nature of the issues that are being raised. Issues become less urgent and less complex, and they feel less out of control. The aim of counselling should always be to put the client in control, to teach them to manage their lives, make their choices and feel empowered and capable.

Counselling should avoid creating any form of dependency, and the control of the session should always be placed firmly in the clients' hands. The most favourable ending is one volunteered by the couple because the need for support is no longer there. The counselling will have reached a natural ending as both partners feel confident that they can manage their relationship together.

RELUCTANCE TO END THE REGULAR SUPPORT

Sometimes, though, we have found that there can be a reluctance to let go of the support that the couple have received from the counselling. If the counsellor feels this is the case, they will need to explore this further with the couple. Sometimes, it may be due to the fear held by the non-autistic partner that once counselling comes to an end, their autistic partner will stop trying, and everything will revert to the way it was before the counselling. This fear is not unfounded; we have both found this to be a very real risk. This fear can be reduced by the offer, if possible, for the couple to return in the future for a one-off counselling session to re-assess their situation and give support to maintain the positive changes they have achieved.

CREATING A TOOLBOX

The autistic partner will already be working hard to fit in socially with friends at work and may have very depleted resources by the time the couple come together in their 'free' time. To try to maintain the same level of effort inside the family home will be near to impossible on a permanent basis and would cause the autistic partner extreme exhaustion, stress and autistic burnout. This is why the toolbox counselling can provide will be particularly important for the non-autistic partner, who will need to be prepared for times when their partner cannot meet their needs. They will need to make room and space for their autistic partner to recharge and rebuild their own resources. Unfortunately, the world does not always cater for the needs of autistic individuals, and daily demands and pressures can all take their toll.

SOCIAL NETWORK

Before counselling comes to an end, the non-autistic partner should be encouraged to build a social support network for themselves and find ways to get their needs met that do not depend on their partner. We are aware that this implies that the non-autistic partner will be doing most of the work, and we are not going to deny that this is frequently the case. It is a fact that some of their partner's needs will be impossible for the autistic partner to meet, no matter how hard they try. It is rarely a case of won't do and is more a case of can't do.

A CHECKLIST

However, it is equally important that the autistic partner continues to make the effort to meet some of their partner's needs, and the counselling should have provided a very strong indication and checklist as to what those needs are. The checklist may include having a fixed time set aside each week devoted to sharing quality time together. This should be put into practice before the counselling ends so that it is already established and in place. The checklist may need to be in a prominent and easily accessible part of the home, frequently consulted by both partners, and multiple copies should be available in case the original is lost.

DISCOVER NEW MUTUAL INTERESTS

The couple should try to find an interest they both share and, if possible, include other people and couples. This could be joining a walking group together, taking part in supporting the environment, such as joining a litter picking group, taking up photography, joining an open water swimming group, or another hobby. This is something that relationship counselling should have explored and once again set in motion before the counselling ends. There are many choices, and if explored enough, at least one hobby or interest will suit both needs.

A BALANCE BETWEEN AUTONOMY AND INTIMACY

What is important is that the strategies that have been shown to be beneficial to both partners and the relationship should be put into place well before the counselling ends and a routine is established. Relationship counselling should explore various ways for the couple to find a balance between autonomy and intimacy that works for both, and this will only be achieved through a process of trial and error. Commitment and hard work will be essential on the part of the couple, and the counsellor will need to be patient and provide ample encouragement to ensure that both partners leave with a toolbox as full as possible.

INCREASING THE TIME BETWEEN SESSIONS

Another reason why there can be reluctance for the couple to withdraw from counselling is that it may feel for one or both partners that they will be cutting off a valuable lifeline that their relationship has come to rely on. A way to help resolve this is to increase the time between sessions slowly. For example, if sessions were weekly, then change them to fortnightly, and when the couple is ready, change them to monthly sessions. The reasons for and usefulness of this will need to be discussed with the couple beforehand, and both will need to consent to the changes. This can feel a little like the weaning process and will encourage clients to become more self-dependent and put into practice the self-help skills they will have learnt in the sessions. In addition, the non-autistic partner should be encouraged to put both emotional and social support systems in place, and they should already benefit from these. This support could be from a support group, finding a hobby to share with others or simply establishing close and dependable links with friends and family who understand their situation.

FOLLOW-UP APPOINTMENT

For the neurodiverse couple, working on the relationship will be constantly ongoing, and if they wish to maintain a healthy relationship, they will need to work on it consistently. They may be concerned about how they will manage new challenges that may evolve in the future. This can be easily remedied by informing the couple that they can return for a one-off session whenever they feel the need is there and the relationship requires some extra maintenance. This could be spaced at three, six or twelve months apart. Sometimes, just knowing that option is there can be enough for the couple, and they will not have the need to pursue it.

PROFESSIONAL GUIDELINES

All counselling governing bodies highlight the importance of appropriate endings in counselling and psychotherapy. The British Association of Counselling and Psychotherapy (2024) offer many useful recommendations on this subject and the importance of getting it right. One of their suggestions is the avoidance of unplanned endings or ending abruptly. This is even more crucial when working with autistic clients, as there will already be a natural avoidance of change and difficulty managing unplanned or unpredictable change.

PREPARATION FOR CLOSURE

If unnecessary anxiety and stress are to be avoided, it is safer to keep endings in mind from the very start of the counselling. Keeping the autistic client aware that at some point, they will not need to attend counselling because they will be in a position to self-manage and have strategies and skills that they can rely on. It will also be important to reiterate that ending the counselling does not mean they cannot return, and unless, for some reason, distance or health prevents them from returning to counselling, the door will remain open to them.

Below we have included a checklist that can be used as a guide to ending counselling sessions and adapted to suit individual clients and couples.

Before Ending Checklist

☐ Introduce the topic of endings from early on in the counselling sessions.

☐ Give ample time for strategies developed in the sessions to be practised.

☐ Give ample time for these strategies to become part of their routine in daily life.

☐ Slowly extend the time between the sessions.

☐ Ensure that both partners feel ready and able to manage alone.

☐ Make as many lists and notes as possible for the couple to take away with them.

☐ Recommend books and journals that may be of use to the couple and provide a reading list.

☐ Give the couple names of any support groups that may be useful to them.

☐ Always let the couple know that they can return to counselling if needed in the future.

☐ Make the boundaries of contact very clear after the counselling has ended.

☐ Make clear that confidentiality will remain with both partners equally after the counselling has ended.

Having clear boundaries regarding what will happen after the relationship counselling has ended is essential, and these should be made very clear and discussed with the couple. Each should receive a written copy of these before the counselling ends. This will be to avoid the confidentiality that is held by the counsellor regarding the couple being challenged. Any correspondence sent should be from both partners. This can only be changed if, in the future, the couple separates, and one partner wishes to return. If this occurs, it will be down to the individual counsellor to decide whether this feels appropriate or if they would be better served by seeking a new counsellor.

REFERRING TO OTHER AGENCIES

Unfortunately, not all relationships can be fixed, and not all partners want their relationship to be fixed. Counsellors are not fairy godmothers and cannot wave a magic wand. Sometimes, couples come to counselling when it is already too late, and the aim of counselling becomes how the couple can best part. This is okay if both partners want the same, and relationship counselling can play an important role in this type of work.

An ending to the counselling may be unavoidable because the counsellor has recognized that their clients' needs are not within their area of expertise. Referring a client or a couple to a suitable service is an ethical duty that all counsellors are responsible for upholding. This could be for psychosexual counselling if sex is the main concern. It maybe referring onto mediation services, if the couple wish to separate and there are children involved or strong issues that counselling cannot resolve. If there is an addiction or a mental health concern, then referring to someone who specializes in that area would be more appropriate. It is vital that a counsellor can recognize when they should refer a couple on, which should be carried out very sensitively. Always discuss working with neurodiverse couples in supervision. Ensure that the supervisor is also trained or experienced in this area of expertise. This will be very helpful in identifying when a referral should be recommended to a couple or individual.

IN CONCLUSION

The idea for this book first began in 2014. We both decided that the only way to discover what neurodiverse couples needed from relationship counselling was to ask them. To uncover what they had experienced first-hand and to learn from that experience and act on their recommendations for ways relationship counselling could be improved. Being understood proved to be an overwhelming factor in the success of the therapeutic relationship and the outcome of the counselling.

This international research has highlighted the need for all relationship counsellors to receive adequate training in working with autistic neurodiversity. We hope this book will help us achieve that aim. Unfortunately, many neurodiverse couples have been severely let down by the counselling they have received. Consequently, couples and families have fallen apart, impacting not just the couple but, in many cases, their children and the whole family system.

Our survey and other research has highlighted the difficulty couples have experienced in trying to find a relationship counsellor trained in autism and neurodiverse romantic relationships (Holmes, 2023; Smith et al., 2020). Holmes describes how the participants in their study stated they had to see between five and seven counsellors before finding a counsellor who was trained and experienced in autism and neurodiversity. Smith et al. reported that the interviewees in their research study found the same difficulty due to a lack of knowledge and training to work in this area.

Neurodiverse couples deserve the best possible chance that counselling services can provide, and now that there is a wealth of information available, there is no reason or excuse for this not to be the case. We both thank you for taking the time to read this book and for developing your understanding of what it means to be in a neurodiverse relationship and work with neurodiverse couples. We would like to end with the two quotes below, the first from a female non-autistic partner and the second from a male autistic partner. Both show the benefits that can come out of relationship counselling when the counsellor is adequately trained and experienced:

(NAFP) 'The counsellor saved our marriage... I thought he (autistic partner) had schizophrenia or multiple personalities. I could not make sense of it. Our counsellor validated me and made me feel worthy of a good relationship. I loved him but was scared because I didn't know how to help him. The diagnosis helped show him I loved him in a way he could understand. It gave me the resources to do my own research and to ask him the right questions... It saved our marriage'.

(AMP) 'She helped us communicate and better understand each other. She helped me address some issues from my past which were sensitive to my partner. She helped us cope during a period when my partner had a very hectic job, and we were living in a place I struggled to cope with'.

REFERENCES

British Association of Counselling and Psychotherapy. (2024). *Endings: What complaints tell us*. www.bacp.co.uk/about-us/protecting-the-public/professional-conduct/what-complaints-tell-us/endings

Holmes, S. (2023). Exploring a later in life diagnosis and its impact on marital satisfaction in the lost generation of autistic adults: An exploratory phenomenological qualitative study. *Global Journal of Intellectual & Developmental Disabilities, 12*. doi:10.19080/GJIDD.2023.12.555829.

Smith, R., Netto, J., Gribble, N., & Falkmer, M. (2020). 'At the end of the day, it's love': An exploration of relationships in neurodiverse couples. *Journal of Autism and Developmental Disorders, 51*(9), 3311–3321. doi:10.1007/s10803-020-04790-z.

Appendix 1: Questionnaire

IS COUPLE COUNSELLING USEFUL WHEN ONE PARTNER IS ON THE AUTISM SPECTRUM?

Maxine Aston MSc and Professor Tony Attwood

1. Have you been for couple counselling?

2. Are you or your partner autistic?

If you answered yes to both of the above and would be willing to take the time to complete a questionnaire then please click the link below. Once you have completed the questionnaire then please return to _____.

The aim of the research is to provide a better understanding of how therapists may best support couples when one partner is autistic.

You have the right to withdraw your information and it will not be used in the research.

The information you provide may be used for research and possibly publication. We will remove any identifying information. You have the right to remain anonymous.

SECTION 1 - INFORMATION ABOUT YOU

- Name (optional)
- Contact information (optional)
- Your age
- Your nationality
- Your religion
- Your occupation

- Your highest academic qualification

- Your relationship status

- Is your relationship ongoing?

- Length of the relationship

- Length of marriage or civil partnership

- Have you been diagnosed with Asperger's syndrome or an autism spectrum disorder?

SECTION 2 - INFORMATION ABOUT YOUR PARTNER

- Their age

- Their nationality

- Their religion

- Their occupation

- Their highest academic qualification

- Have they been diagnosed as autistic, Asperger's syndrome or autism spectrum disorder?

- If YES when?

- Have they completed the AS Quotient?

- If yes what was their score?

QUESTIONNAIRE SET 1

1. When did you attend counselling?

2. How long did you attend for?

3. How did you find your therapist or counsellor?

4. Was your therapist male or female?

5. Were they aware you or your partner is autistic?

6. Were they trained to work in this area?

7. Do you know what type of therapy they offered? For example CBT, psychodynamic?

8. What was the most useful aspect of the counselling?

9. What was the least useful aspect of the counselling?

10. Do you believe the counselling had a positive effect on the relationship?

11. If yes, what were the positive effects on yourself?

12. If yes, what were the positive effects on your partner?

13. Do you feel the counselling had a negative effect on the relationship?

14. If yes, what were the negative effects on yourself?

15. If yes, what were the negative effects on your partner?

16. Would you attend couple counselling in the future?

17. How could current relationship counselling be improved when a partner is autistic?

In your own words please describe your experience of couple counselling.

Appendix 2: Autistic Respondents and Their Partners

Autistic Respondents	Partners of Autistic Respondents
Average Age: 49 Years Age Span: 28–70 Years	Average Age: 45 Years Age Span: 26–82 Years

Average Length of Relationship: 19 Years
Span of 2–42 Years

Autistic Respondents	N=41	Partners of Autistic Respondents	N=41
Male	25	Male	17
Female	16	Female	24
		Non-autistic	37
		Autistic	4

Nationality		Nationality	
British	26	British	27
American	7	American	5
Australian	1	Australian	1
New Zealand	1	New Zealand	2
Canadian	1	Canadian	1
Belgian	1	Belgian	1
Black British	0	Black British	1

Autistic Respondents	N=41	Partners of Autistic Respondents	N=41
Japanese	0	Japanese	1
Russian	0	Russian	1
Irish	0	Irish	1
German	1	German	0
Greek	1	Greek	0
Dutch	1	Dutch	0
Italian	1	Italian	0

Occupations		Occupations	
Engineering	7	Homemakers	9
Military & Government	6	Health Care	7
IT	4	Teachers	4
Retired/Unemployed	3	Counsellors	3
Architecture	3	Director/Manager	3
Legal Profession	2	Clerical	2
Nursing	2	Architecture	2
Accountancy	1	Accountant	1
Translator	1	Priest	1
Dentistry	1	Gardener	1
Vet	1	Not known	8
GP	1		
Professional Driver	1		
Psychologist/Therapist	1		
Balloon Pilot	1		
Priest	1		
Unemployed	1		
Not known	4		

Appendix 3: Non-Autistic Respondents and Their Autistic Partners

Non-Autistic Respondents	Autistic Partners of Non-Autistic Respondents
Average Age: 50 Years **Age Span: 23–74 Years**	**Average Age: 52 Years** **Age Span: 19–75 Years**

Average Length of Relationship: 21 Years
Span of 2–50 Years

Non-Autistic Respondents	N=184	Autistic Partners of Non-Autistic Respondents	N=184
Male	4	Male	5
Female	174	Female	173
Not known	6	Not known	6

Nationality		Nationality	
British	60	British	61
American	57	American	55
Australian	25	Australian	24
Canadian	7	Canadian	7
German	4	German	1
New Zealand	3	New Zealand	5
Dutch	2	Dutch	5

Non-Autistic Respondents	N=184	Autistic Partners of Non-Autistic Respondents	N=184
South African	2	South African	1
Swedish	1	Swedish	0
Belgian	1	Belgian	1
Dominican	1	Dominican	0
Zimbabwean	1	Zimbabwean	1
Mexican	1	Mexican	0
Irish	1	Irish	0
Anglo-Irish	1	Anglo-Irish	0
Hungarian	1	Hungarian	0
Not known	16	Not known	14
Danish	0	Danish	1
Japanese	0	Japanese	1
Scottish	0	Scottish	1
Scottish/Spanish	0	Scottish/Spanish	1
Indian	0	Indian	1
Ugandan	0	Ugandan	1
Asian	0	Asian	1
Black American	0	Black American	1
Spanish	0	Spanish	1

Occupations		Occupations	
Teaching	23	Engineering	30
Counsellor/Therapist	22	IT	20
Homemaker/Mother	19	Retired	20
Nursing	13	Managerial	15
Psychologist	9	Teacher/trainer	8
Retired	9	Accountant	6

Writer/Journalist	5	Medical	5
Carers	5	Architect	3
Administration	5	Musician	3
Sales	6	Share Trader / Investor	3
Pathologist / Speech & Language	4	Clergy	2
Psychiatrist	4	Dentist	2
Consultant	4	Clerical	2
Director	4	Farmer	2
Academic	3	Driver	2
Researcher	3	Chemistry Adjunct	1
Self-Employed	3	Government	1
Dietician	2	Cartographer	1
Dental Hygienist	2	Not known	58
Engineering	2		
Not known	37		

Appendix 4: Would You Attend Couple Counselling in the Future?

AUTISTIC RESPONDENTS

- Out of 41 respondents, 26 (63.4%) answered Yes (one stated – but not with Relate. Another stated his wife won't attend).

- Out of these 26 respondents, 16 (61.5%) stated they would only attend if the counsellor was trained, knowledgeable or experienced in working with autism and autistic/non-autistic couples.

- Out of 41 respondents, 7 (17%) said No.

- Out of 41 respondents, 8 (19.5%) were unsure.

NON-AUTISTIC RESPONDENTS

- Out of 184 respondents, 176 (95.6%) gave an answer to this question.

- Out of these 176 respondents, 96 (54.5%) answered Yes.

- Out of these 96 respondents who answered Yes, 50 (52%) said they would only attend if the counsellor was trained, knowledgeable or experienced in working with autism and autistic/non-autistic couples. (Out of these 50 respondents, 3 said they would only go if they could see Tony or Maxine and 1 said only if they had read Maxine's book.)

- Out of the 176 respondents, 14 (8%) said they would go but their partner would not or would need to change first.

- Out of the 176 respondents, 41 (23.3%) said they would not go to counselling again.

- Out of the 176 respondents, 16 (9%) were not sure if they would seek couple counselling again.

- Out of the 176 respondents, 9 (5.1%) were presently attending couple counselling.

Subject Index

Author Index

Adams, S. 176
American Association of Marriage and
Family Therapy (AAMFT) 38–9
American Psychiatric Association
(APA) 79, 110, 219
Anders, S. 130
Anderson, J. R. 213
Arad, P. 63, 91, 93, 108, 113
Asakura, T. 54, 59, 62, 113, 114
Aston, M. 93, 108, 133, 146, 150, 163,
164, 166, 167, 193, 201, 206
Attwood, T. 17, 53, 91, 166, 174

Bagby, R. M. 102
Bancroft, J. 165
Barnett, J. P. 163
Baron-Cohen, S. 36, 87, 144
Beach, S. R. H. 111
Bentley, K. 108
Bergin, A. E. 28
Bird, G. 84
Bishop-Fitzpatrick, L. 176
Bolling, K. M. 94, 95
Bostock-Ling, J. 113
Bougeard, C. 177
Brede, J. 174
British Association of Counselling and
Psychotherapy (BACP) 37, 55, 229
Brodley, B. T. 31
Brosnan, M. 176
Brown, J. 87
Butwicka, A. 176

Cage, E. 151
Camm-Crosbie, L. 70

Çapri, B. 111
Cardon, G. 158
Carson-Wong, A. 44
Cassidy, S. 30, 173
Cazalis, F. 166
Centers for Disease Control
and Prevention 79
Chapman, G. 50, 140, 205
Cheung, A. 177
Choi, H. 108
Cooper, K. 37
Crompton, C. J. 129, 130, 136, 158

DeBrabander, K. M. 33
Deguchi, N. 54, 59, 62, 113, 114
Durmuş, E. 111

English, M. 87
Evans, C. 172, 173

Feldman, G. C. 63
Fernandes, L. C. 166
Ferri, P. 111
Fletcher-Watson, S. 84

Gable, S. L. 145
Garnett, M. 174
Geurts, H. M. 172, 177
Gibbs, V. 155
Gillis, J. M. 18
Gillott, A. 37
Gökçakan, Z. 111
Gotham, K. 91
Gottman, J. M. 147

Tudor, K. 31
Turner, D. 165, 166

Ustundag-Budak, M. 44

Vivanti, G. 177

Warburton, W. A. 93
Wilson, B. 96, 108, 112, 113, 114, 132, 141

Yew, R. Y. 130, 162